Somatic Therapy for Seniors

Healing Paths for Stress Reduction, Trauma Recovery and Renewed Well-Being

Table of Contents

Introduction............................7

Chapter 1: Understanding Somatic Therapy 11

What Is Somatic Therapy?11

Types of Somatic Therapies 12

Principle of Somatic Therapy 14

Mind-Body Connection............... 14

Sensory Awareness 14

Embodied Presence 14

Trauma-Informed Approach 15

Movement and Expression 15

Regulation and Integration 15

Holistic Approach 15

Relevance to Seniors 16

Physical Health Benefits 16

Stress Reduction 16

Emotional Well-Being 17

Pain Management........................17

Improved Quality of Life 17

Historical Context 18

Chapter 2: The Impact of Stress on Seniors 21

Physical and Mental Effects 22

Physical Effects 22

Mental Effects 23

Common Stressors in Aging 24

Importance of Stress Reduction for Well-Being 26

How Stress Affects The Body And Mind 27

Benefits of Stress Reduction 27

Physical Health 27

Mental Health 28

Improved Cognitive Function.....28

Better Sleep Quality 28

Enhanced Resilience...................28

Improved Relationships 29

Increased Enjoyment of Life.......29

Chapter 3: Trauma in Later Life 30

Types of Trauma Seniors May Experience................31

Interpersonal Trauma................. 31

Historical Trauma....................... 31

Medical Trauma.........................32

Loss and Bereavement................32

Natural Disasters 32

Community Violence 32

Discrimination and Marginalization...........................33

Financial Exploitation 33

Isolation and Loneliness............33

Recognizing Trauma Symptoms.........................33

Emotional Symptoms 34

Physical Symptoms.....................34

Behavioral Symptoms.................35

Cognitive Symptoms 36

Relational Symptoms 36

The Role of Somatic Therapy in Trauma Healing *37*

Chapter 4: Somatic Approaches to Stress Reduction **39**

Mind-Body Connection ... 40

Breathwork and Relaxation Techniques *41*

Ideas for Getting Started 42

Biodynamic Breathwork 43

Part 1 43

Part 2 45

Part 3 45

Holotropic Breathwork 47

The Wim Hof Method 48

Tips 49

Progressive Muscle Relaxation *49*

Visualization *51*

Self-Massage *52*

Mindfulness Meditation ... *54*

Rhythmic Movement and Mindful Exercise *55*

Tips *55*

Integrating Breathwork With Movement *56*

Diaphragmatic Breathing 56

Laughter Yoga 58

Vinyasa Yoga 59

Tips 61

Chapter 5: Mindful Movement Sequences 62

Here's a Simple Mindful Movement Sequence *62*

Fluid Transitions Between Exercises *64*

Here's How to Do It 66

Seated, Standing, and Lying Down Exercises *67*

Seated Exercises 67

Seated Forward Fold (Paschimottanasana) 68

Seated Twist (Ardha Matsyendrasana) 69

Thunderbolt Pose (Vajrasana) 69

Standing Exercises 70

Sideways Bending Pose (Konasana) 70

Chair Pose (Utkatasana) 71

Tree Pose (Vrksasana) 71

Lying Down Exercises 72

Corpse Pose (Savasana) 72

Supine Twist 73

Bridge Pose (Setu Bandhasana) . 73

Personalization and Adaptations *74*

Personalization 74

Adaptation 76

Chapter 6: Practical Somatic Exercises for Seniors **79**

Diverse Range of Exercises *80*

Calming Breathing Technique... 80

Breathing While In Pain 82

Chinese Breathing........................83

Neck Rolls 84

Seated Resistance Band
Exercises 85

Qigong...87

Body Scan Meditation.................89

Interactive Elements 91

Variety and Creativity 92

*Progressive Exercises for
Strength and Flexibility ...94*

Some Exercises for Strength and
Flexibility 95

Lunge With a Spinal Twist..........95

Forward Fold...............................96

Triceps Stretch 98

Bodyweight Squat 100

Push-Up 101

Plank 103

**Chapter 7: Integrating
Breathwork Into Somatic
Practices 105**

*Breathing Exercises for
Relaxation 107*

Box Breathing 107

Equal Breathing 108

Deep Breathing 109

Tips 110

*Syncing Breath With
Movements 111*

*How to Sync Breath With
Movement........................112*

During Inhalation 113

Inhale at the Top and Hold Your
Breath on the Way Down...........113

Inhale Throughout the Entire
Descent......................................113

During Exhalation......................113

Exhaling at the Bottom or
Throughout the Movement........114

Holding the Breath Throughout
the Movement 114

*Mindful Breathing for Stress
Reduction........................114*

Breath Awareness Meditation ...115

Pursed-Lip Breathing 117

Mindful Slow and Deep
Breathing...................................118

Tips 119

**Chapter 8: Building a
Community Through
Somatic Practices....... 120**

*Group Participation
Exercises 121*

Body Scan Meditation.............. 122

Partner Stretching.................... 122

Mirror Exercises ....

Group Breathing Exercises 122

Guided Movement
Exploration 123

Circle Sharing........................... 123

Grounding and Centering
Practices 123

Some Group Exercises ...124

Partner Forward Fold 124

Four-Person Plank.................... 125

Temple Pose............................. 127

Partner Boat Pose 128

Fostering Connection and Shared Well-Being 129

Feedback Mechanism for Continuous Improvement 130

Chapter 9: Case Studies and Success Stories 133

I. Case Study: John's Journey Towards Healing Through Somatic Therapy 134

Patient's Background 134

Somatic Therapy Approach 134

Treatment Progress 135

Outcome 135

II. Case Study: Lilly's Journey to Healing Through Somatic Therapy 136

Patient Background 136

Somatic Therapy Approach 136

Outcome 137

Real Life Stories 138

Eve's Success Story 138

Mary's Journey to Emotional Healing 139

Thorgal's Success Story 139

Robert's Anxiety Relief 141

Testimonials 142

Outcomes 144

Conclusion 146

Recap of Key Concepts ... 147

I. An Overview of Somatic Therapy for Seniors 147

II. Understanding Somatic Therapy 147

III. Effects of Stress on Seniors 148

IV. Trauma in Later Life 148

V. Somatic Approaches to Stress Reduction 148

VI. Somatic Exercises for E lders 148

VII. Integrating Breathwork With Somatic Practices 149

VIII. Building a Community Through Somatic Practices 149

IX. Case Studies and Success Stories 149

Encouragement for Seniors to Embrace Somatic Healing 149

Resources for Further Exploration 151

References 153

Introduction

Somatic therapy, also known as body psychotherapy, offers a unique approach to healing by recognizing the profound connection between mind and body. It places great importance on the experiences we have in both realms. The very term "somatic" itself encompasses anything related to our physical being, highlighting the holistic nature of this therapeutic method.

Somatic therapy emphasizes the importance of being in tune with our bodies. It entails recognizing the physiological responses triggered by certain stimuli, as well as understanding our bodies reactions throughout the day, like headaches or stomachaches. Developing this awareness plays a crucial role in somatic therapy and leads to better overall well-being (Preskorn & Burke, 1992).

If verbal therapy has reached the limit of its therapeutic potential for a patient, somatic therapy states that the body is a largely unexplored resource for psychotherapy, which we can learn much from. These resources include the gestures, posture, facial expressions, eye gaze, and body movements that may teach us. In addition to talk therapy, somatic therapy practitioners employ mind-body exercises as well as other physical approaches to assist in the release of pent-up stress, which has a detrimental impact on the patient's physical and emotional well-being (Salamon, 2023).

Somatic therapy for seniors is a type of psychotherapy that emphasizes the mind-body link to address emotional, psychological, and physical concerns. This type of therapy acknowledges that experiences and emotions stay not only in the mind but also in the general well-being of seniors who may have collected a lifetime of experiences and physical stressors. Somatic therapy approaches mental health from a holistic point of view, taking into account physical, emotional, cognitive, and spiritual well-being. This approach is especially useful for older people since it acknowledges the multiple aspects of aging and its impact on overall health.

Older people can face physical changes as a result of age, chronic health concerns, or mobility issues. Somatic therapy enables elders to become more aware of their bodies, including sensations, tensions, and areas of discomfort. Seniors who cultivate this awareness will be able to appreciate the links between their bodies and emotional experiences. It frequently includes breathwork and relaxation exercises to assist older people in regulating their neurological systems, reducing stress, and promoting relaxation. Gentle breathing techniques, progressive muscular relaxation, and mindfulness activities can help elderly patients improve their general well-being.

While intensive physical exercise may not be appropriate for seniors, somatic therapy can include light movement routines like stretching, yoga, or tai chi. These activities increase flexibility, mobility, and body awareness while also allowing for emotional expression and release. Through this process, elderly patients can gain insight into their life experiences, develop a deeper connection with themselves, and enhance their overall quality of life. By addressing the mind-body connection and honoring the unique experiences of aging, somatic therapy can empower elderly patients to navigate life transitions with greater ease and grace.

Addressing stress, trauma, and healing in later life is critical for older adults' general well-being. Untreated stress and trauma can increase physical and mental health problems, whereas healing develops resilience and improves quality of life, encouraging emotional, psychological, and physical health in later life. Trauma can have long-term consequences, whether childhood traumas, a big life event, or continuous stress causes it. Unresolved trauma can have a significant influence on our general well-being, influencing our physical health, mental condition, and ability to live fulfilling lives. It is important to recognize the signs and symptoms of unresolved trauma, as well as the relationship between trauma and numerous health disorders.

Trauma can influence your emotional, social, and physical health, so it's critical to address that trauma and deal with it in ways that reduce the impact it has on you subconsciously. Trauma-induced stress can affect your body's stress response system, resulting in an overproduction of stress hormones such as cortisol. This can result in a variety of difficulties, including impaired immune function, inflammation, and an increased chance of acquiring chronic illnesses. Research indicates that persons with a history of trauma are more prone to acquire autoimmune diseases, cardiovascular issues, chronic pain, and gastrointestinal difficulties. When we heal from previous trauma, we shed the weight that has been holding us back. It's like taking off a heavy burden that restricts your movement.

By digesting our experiences and emotions, we obtain a better understanding of ourselves and learn coping methods that will help us face future obstacles. There is no one-size-fits-all approach to healing from past traumas. However, therapy is a widely used and effective treatment. Therapy with a qualified expert can give us a secure environment in which to explore and process our traumas. Somatic therapy is one of many therapeutic modalities available to meet the specific needs of each individual. Accepting the healing process enables us to reclaim our lives, achieve inner peace, and lay the groundwork for a healthier and happier existence (Dugan, 24 C.E.).

Chapter 1: Understanding Somatic Therapy

What Is Somatic Therapy?

Somatic therapy, commonly known as somatic experiencing (SE) therapy, is a novel type of psychotherapy created by Peter Levine, Ph.D., a psychotherapist and founder of Somatic Experiencing International. Somatic techniques focus primarily on the body rather than the mind (Krouse, 2023). "It's a treatment focusing on the body and how emotions appear within the body". "Somatic therapies believe that unresolved emotional issues can become 'trapped' inside" (Salamon, 2023).

Somatic experience therapy treats chronic and post-traumatic stress by emphasizing bodily awareness over thoughts and emotions. SE is frequently referred to as a bottom-up strategy for treating trauma-related disorders. While talk therapy focuses on thoughts and feelings that occur in the "higher" portions of the brain, SE begins by probing the more "primitive" parts of the brain.

SE adheres to the basis that trauma is stored inside your body and mind. Following a terrifying or upsetting encounter, some people may develop a maladaptive stress response. In this instance, the body's alert system becomes "stuck" in an overactive condition. Somatic experience practitioners think that physical movement, such as slight shaking and posture modifications, can facilitate a bodily "release" that promotes healing and recovery. Recognizing and discussing physical experiences may help to restore nervous system balance (Krouse, 2023).

Types of Somatic Therapies

There are many types of somatic therapy. Some of them are under

1. Alexander Technique

The Alexander Technique teaches people how to move in a more balanced and coordinated manner.

2. Feldenkrais Method

The Feldenkrais Method uses gentle movements and touches to assist people in becoming more aware of their body's movement patterns.

3. Hatha Yoga

Hatha yoga is a type of yoga that emphasizes physical positions, or asanas, and breathwork.

4. Iyengar Yoga

Iyengar yoga is a hatha yoga style in which supports are used to assist students in performing poses.

5. Pilates

Pilates is a mat-based workout regimen that focuses on strength, flexibility, and balance.

6. Qigong

Qigong is an ancient Chinese exercise that combines gentle movements with focused breathing.

7. Rolfing

Rolfing is a type of deep-tissue massage technique that focuses on realigning the muscles, fascia, organs, bones, and nerves to improve posture. This can help people relax in their bodies by alleviating any pain they may be feeling.

8. Somatic yoga

Somatic yoga mixes traditional hatha yoga with somatic practices to calm the mind while strengthening the body.

9. Tai Chi Chuan

Tai Chi Chuan is an internal martial art discipline that uses meditation-like movement patterns at modest speeds (often less than 70 beats per minute). People who frequently practice tai chi are urged to connect with their spiritual selves.

10. Yoga Nidra

Yoga Nidra is a guided meditation that calms the body and mind. It can assist in reducing tension, stress, and anxiety.

Principle of Somatic Therapy

Somatic therapy is based on many key principles that highlight the mutual dependence of the body and mind, as well as the value of bodily sensations in psychological rehabilitation. Here are some important principles of somatic therapy.

Mind-Body Connection

Somatic treatment acknowledges that the body and mind have an unbreakable connection, with psychological difficulties manifesting as physical symptoms and vice versa. Using body sensations and experiences, therapists assist clients in accessing and processing underlying emotions and psychological patterns.

Sensory Awareness

Clients are guided to become more aware of bodily sensations like tension, relaxation, pain, and pleasure. They learn to tune into their body, have a better understanding of themselves, and regulate their emotions through mindfulness techniques and sensory awareness activities.

Embodied Presence

Somatic treatment emphasizes the value of being completely present in one's body and experiencing the moment. Therapists teach clients to create embodied presence through grounding techniques, breathwork, and somatic experiences, resulting in a stronger connection with themselves and their surroundings.

Trauma-Informed Approach

Somatic therapists use a trauma-informed approach, which acknowledges the influence of past traumas on clients' physical and mental health. They provide a secure and supportive setting for clients to examine and process their traumatic experiences, fostering healing and resilience.

Movement and Expression

Somatic treatment relies heavily on movement and expressive strategies. Therapists may use gentle movement, dancing, yoga, or other expressive arts techniques to assist clients in releasing physical tension, expressing emotions, and accessing deeper layers of embodied experience.

Regulation and Integration

Somatic therapy aims to regulate the nervous system and integrate different components of the self. Clients learn how to manage their physiological responses, integrate mind-body experiences, and enhance overall well-being by using techniques including breathwork, relaxation, and mindfulness.

Holistic Approach

Somatic therapy provides a comprehensive approach to

healing, recognizing the interconnection of the physical, emotional, mental, and spiritual dimensions of health. Therapists address the requirements of their clients holistically, assisting them on their journey toward greater wholeness, balance, and vitality.

Relevance to Seniors

As life expectancy keeps on rising in industrialized countries, so will the incidence of emotional and mental problems like depression among seniors. The good news is that there are numerous successful therapy approaches and activities for improving resilience in seniors. Somatic therapy can be pretty relevant and beneficial to seniors for a variety of reasons (Lonczak, 2021).

Physical Health Benefits

Somatic therapy frequently incorporates movement-based techniques like yoga, tai chi, and mild stretching exercises. These techniques can help seniors enhance their flexibility, strength, balance, and overall physical well-being, which is especially important as we age and these abilities deteriorate.

Stress Reduction

Many seniors experience more significant stress as a result of health difficulties, the loss of loved ones, or changes in their living arrangements. Somatic therapy approaches, such as deep breathing exercises or body scans, can assist seniors in lowering stress while improving their ability to deal with everyday challenges.

Emotional Well-Being

Somatic therapy focuses on the mind-body link, acknowledging that emotional and psychological difficulties can appear as physical symptoms. By concentrating on bodily sensations and movement, seniors can become more aware of and process their emotions, resulting in better emotional health and well-being.

Pain Management

Chronic pain is frequent among seniors and may substantially influence the quality of life. Somatic therapy approaches, such as gentle movement and body awareness exercises, can assist seniors with pain management, tension reduction, and overall comfort.

Improved Quality of Life

Somatic therapy can improve seniors' quality of life by enhancing their physical and mental health. It can help them stay active, engaged, and connected to their bodies and emotions, resulting in a stronger sense of vitality and satisfaction.

Overall, somatic therapy provides elders with a comprehensive approach to health and well-being, addressing the interdependence of mind, body, and spirit. It can be a successful strategy for seniors who want to improve their physical health, mental well-being, and general quality of life.

Historical Context

Somatic therapy has a long history in psychology, medicine, and philosophy, emerging as a unique field in the 20th century. However, its roots can be traced back to ancient traditions and philosophical ideas about the mind-body link. Ancient civilizations, such as the Greeks and Egyptians, recognized the link between physical and mental health, as seen in practices like yoga and meditation.

In the 19th century, pioneers like Wilhelm Wundt, William James, and Sigmund Freud laid the foundation for bodily therapy with their work on the unconscious mind and the body's role in psychological processes. The early 20th century saw the rise of somatic pioneers such as F.M. Alexander, Moshe Feldenkrais, and Elsa Gindler, who emphasized body awareness and movement in health. As somatic principles integrated into mainstream psychology and medicine in the mid-20th century, figures like Wilhelm Reich and Alexander Lowen developed body-centered psychotherapy approaches.

Somatics evolved as a field due to various experiences involving the living body, such as disease, physical restrictions, and exposure to new practices. Pioneers realized that deep listening to the body can heal and enhance movement and vitality. This revolution in understanding the body corresponded with a societal transformation that deviated from Victorian norms. Somatics, influenced by theorists like Dewey and Merleau-

Ponty, emerged as a recognized approach to experiential learning and sensory research, providing new methods to engage with and comprehend the body. The somatic inquiry was boosted by the rise of existentialism and empirical research, as well as by dance and expressionism. The pioneering work of Freud, Jung, and Reich in psychology, Delsartes, Laban, and Dalcroze in cultural studies (art, architecture, crystallography, dance, and music), Heinrich Jacoby and John Dewey in education, and Edmond Jacobson in medical research propelled these developments into new frontiers. New methods of physical care and education arose as a result of the unique experiences of exploratory individuals all over the world. However, it took some 50 years for scholars to recognize this phenomenon as a single field of somatic education.

Thomas Hanna, Don Hanlon Johnson, and Seymour Kleinman recognized similarities in the methodologies of somatic pioneers such as Gerda Alexander, F.M. Alexander, Feldenkrais, Gindler, Laban, Mensendieck, Middendorf, Mézières, Rolf, Todd, and Trager, as well as their protégés. These techniques stress breathing, sensation, and listening to the body, frequently beginning with conscious relaxation. To better understand oneself, students are instructed to focus on their physiological feelings and move gently. Proprioceptive signals were stimulated using both skilled touch and verbal stimulation. Eastern beliefs and practices, such as yoga and martial arts, influenced somatic techniques. These pioneers' work formed a canon of exercises, concepts, and inquiry systems now used in educational programs worldwide. The somatic inquiry has also made its way into research approaches such as action research, ethnographic studies, and phenomenology.

Hanna delivered the term somatics in the 1970s to characterize and group these processes together. Philosophers and scholars from the late 20th century collaborated to shape the new area of Somatic Education. Mangione (1993) outlines how the global communication explosion and cultural upheavals of the 1970s resulted in a true boom in somatics. The somatic world has three branches: somatic psychology, somatic bodywork, and somatic movement (Eddy 2004). Dance professionals have contributed significantly to advancing bodily movement and the discipline of Somatic Movement Education and Therapy (SME&T). SME&T entails listening to the body and reacting to these sensations by intentionally changing movement patterns and choices.

Dance has catalyzed the research of movement expression and somatic education, resulting in the emergence of various somatic disciplines. Many somatic pioneers, notably Bartenieff, started as dancers, bringing a thorough grasp of movement to their somatic practices. Through inward exploration and exposure to cultures that value introspection, these leaders created novel ways to move and engage. Their work, including Bartenieff's Fundamentals, has dramatically impacted both the somatic and dance worlds, helping to bridge the gap between somatic instruction and artistic expression.

In recent decades, somatic therapy has grown to include new approaches such as Hakomi Therapy and Sensorimotor Psychotherapy, which emphasize the body's involvement in trauma healing and emotional regulation. Overall, somatic therapy takes a holistic approach to health, recognizing the interdependence of mind, body, and spirit in healing (Eddy, 2009).

Chapter 2: The Impact of Stress on Seniors

Stress can substantially impact seniors' health, affecting many elements of their well-being. One of the fundamental effects of stress is that it weakens the immune system, making older people more vulnerable to conditions like colds, the flu, and infections. This reduced immune response can also slow the healing process, making it harder to recover from health issues.

Furthermore, stress is strongly linked to heart problems in seniors. When stressed, the body produces adrenaline, which increases blood pressure and heart rate. Over time, this can contribute to the development of heart disease, increasing the likelihood of heart attacks and strokes. Stress can also trigger unhealthy coping behaviors, such as binge drinking, overeating, or drug use—all of which can harm the heart and circulatory system.

In addition, persistent stress might impair seniors' vision and hearing: Long-term adrenaline can restrict small blood vessels, causing temporary hearing and vision impairments. Stress can also cause digestive problems because it triggers the body's "fight or flight" response, which disrupts regular digestive processes. This can cause symptoms including constipation, diarrhea, heartburn, and, in extreme cases, can lead to irritable bowel syndrome and ulcers.

Stress can also harm seniors' dental health as they may unwittingly clench or grind their teeth in response to stress. This can raise the risk of fractures, cavities, and other dental issues. Stress can also promote inflammation in the stomach and intestines, resulting in gastrointestinal pain and problems such as an upset stomach.

Given these concerns, managing stress is critical for seniors. Somatic therapy, regular exercise, a good diet, relaxation techniques, and social support are all effective ways for seniors to reduce stress and improve their overall health and well-being. Addressing stress and its impacts can help seniors maintain better physical and mental health as they age (HCA DEV, 2019).

Physical and Mental Effects

Stress can have various physical and mental impacts on individuals, affecting their current and long-term health. Here are some of the main effects.

Physical Effects

- **Immune system:** Chronic stress can impair the immune system, leaving the body more vulnerable to infections and disorders.

- **Cardiovascular health:** Stress can lead to high blood pressure, heart disease, heart attacks, and strokes.

- **Digestive system:** Stress can cause stomach aches, bloating, diarrhea, and other digestive problems. It can also worsen illnesses such as irritable bowel syndrome.

- **Musculoskeletal system:** Stress can create muscle

tension, resulting in headaches, backaches, stiffness, and pain.

- **Reproductive system:** Women's menstrual cycles and fertility might be affected by stress. In men, it can cause erectile dysfunction and lower testosterone levels.

- **Skin:** Stress can aggravate skin disorders, including acne, eczema, and psoriasis. It can also cause hair loss.

- **Weight changes:** Some people may eat more or less when stressed, resulting in weight increase or reduction.

Mental Effects

- **Anxiety:** Stress can cause or exacerbate anxiety problems, resulting in excessive worry, restlessness, and difficulty concentrating.

- **Depression:** Chronic stress can contribute to the development of depression, which is defined by feelings of melancholy, hopelessness, and loss of interest in activities.

- **Cognitive function:** Stress can affect memory, focus, and decision-making skills.

- **Sleep disturbances:** Stress can cause insomnia, restless sleep, and other sleeping difficulties.

- **Mood changes:** Stress can lead to mood fluctuations, irritation, and feeling overwhelmed.

- **Substance abuse:** Substance abuse can occur when people use alcohol, drugs, or other substances to cope with stress.

Overall, persistent stress can have severe consequences on

both our physical and mental health. To lessen the harmful impacts of stress on our well-being, we should discover healthy ways to handle it, such as through exercise, relaxation techniques, therapy, and social support.

Common Stressors in Aging

Stressors that adults commonly experience can vary depending on their circumstances. However, some universal stressors exist:

- **Work-related stress:** Work-related stress can arise from various factors such as job insecurity, long working hours, tight deadlines, conflicts with coworkers or supervisors, or dissatisfaction with the job.

- **Financial stress:** Financial stress can stem from concerns about income, debts, bills, or future savings and can be a significant source of stress for many adults.

- **Relationship issues:** Relationship issues can also cause significant stress, particularly in cases where there are problems with romantic partners, family members, or friends. These problems include conflicts, communication issues, or significant life changes such as separation or divorce.

- **Health concern:** Dealing with illness, chronic pain, or disabilities can be highly stressful, as can caring for sick or elderly family members.

- **Major life changes:** Life changes such as moving, getting married, having children, or experiencing significant loss can be stressful as they require adapting to new circumstances.

- **Loss of loved ones:** As individuals age, they are likely to experience the loss of several friends and acquaintances. This can lead to concerns about their health and lifespan, as well as feelings of sadness and depression. The stress of worrying about losing close friends can be an everyday occurrence. If your loved one does lose someone close to them, it can be helpful if you understand the grief process and offer a supportive shoulder to lean on when needed.

- **Loneliness:** As individuals age, they may experience different changes in life, such as the loss of loved ones. This can cause a sense of loneliness, which can be more intense if changes like losing a close friend, a spouse, or the inability to drive result in reduced interactions with other people. Less social interaction can lead to isolation and loneliness, which can cause significant stress.

- **Trauma and past experiences:** Past trauma, whether from childhood or adulthood, can have long-lasting effects on mental health if left unaddressed.

- **Social pressure:** Expectations from society, cultural norms, or perceived judgments from others can create stress as individuals try to meet or exceed these expectations.

- **Lack of self-care:** Neglecting physical and mental health needs, such as poor diet, lack of exercise, insufficient sleep, or ignoring emotional well-being, can lead to chronic stress.

Recognizing these stressors and developing healthy coping

mechanisms to manage them effectively is essential. Seeking support from friends, family, or mental health professionals can also be beneficial in navigating stressors (KIM, 2020) (Heydlauf, 2023).

Importance of Stress Reduction for Well-Being

Stress reduction is essential for total well-being because it directly affects our physical, emotional, and mental health. Persistent stress can have a variety of negative consequences, including an increased risk of chronic diseases such as heart disease, obesity, and diabetes, as well as the worsening of mental health issues such as anxiety and depression. Furthermore, high stress levels may affect cognitive function, memory, and decision-making skills. Individuals can improve their quality of life, increase resilience, and build a sense of peace and balance by actively managing stress using approaches such as mindfulness, exercise, relaxation techniques, and seeking social support. Prioritizing stress reduction benefits physical health and promotes emotional stability, healthier relationships, and overall life fulfillment.

How Stress Affects The Body And Mind

It's pronounced that minimizing stress in your daily life will make you happier and healthier. But what makes stress such an effective predictor of overall well-being in the first place? Let's look at how stress affects the body and mind and how stress management can help you enhance your mood, strengthen your immune function, and live longer.

When you are worried, your brain undergoes chemical and physical changes that impair its general function. During times of high stress, some chemicals in the brain, such as the neurotransmitters dopamine, adrenaline, and norepinephrine, begin to increase, resulting in higher levels of these and other "fight-or-flight" hormones. Releasing these substances has physiological effects such as increased heart rate, blood pressure, and a weakened immune system. Stress can cause a variety of mental and emotional illnesses, including anxiety, phobias, and panic attacks, in addition to its physical effects (Eliaz, 2011).

Benefits of Stress Reduction

Stress reduction is important for overall well-being for several reasons.

Physical Health

By reducing stress, individuals can lower their risk of developing numerous physical health problems, including heart disease, high blood pressure, obesity, diabetes, and weakened immune function. It can also promote better physical health.

Mental Health

Persistent stress can take a toll on mental well-being, contributing to anxiety, depression, irritability, mood swings, and other mental health issues. Stress reduction techniques, such as mindfulness, meditation, and relaxation exercises, can help alleviate these symptoms and promote better mental health.

Improved Cognitive Function

High stress levels can impair cognitive function, including memory, concentration, and decision-making abilities. By reducing stress, individuals can enhance their cognitive performance and productivity in various aspects of life, including work, school, and personal relationships.

Better Sleep Quality

Stress often interferes with sleep, leading to difficulty falling, staying, or experiencing restorative sleep. By managing stress effectively, individuals can improve their sleep quality and overall energy levels, leading to better physical and mental functioning throughout the day.

Enhanced Resilience

Learning how to cope with stress in healthy ways can build resilience and the ability to bounce back from adversity and adapt to challenging situations. By developing resilience, individuals can navigate life's ups and downs more effectively and maintain a sense of well-being despite stressors.

Improved Relationships

Chronic stress can strain relationships with family members, friends, and romantic partners due to increased irritability, conflicts, and emotional distancing. Individuals can strengthen their relationships and foster greater connection and support by reducing stress and learning effective communication and conflict-resolution skills.

Increased Enjoyment of Life

Excessive stress can dampen enjoyment and satisfaction, making it difficult to appreciate the present moment and engage in activities that bring joy and fulfillment. By prioritizing stress reduction and practicing self-care, individuals can enhance their overall quality of life and find greater happiness and contentment (Moore, 2022)(Eliaz, 2011).

Chapter 3: Trauma in Later Life

Trauma at any stage of life can have a significant impact on a person's mental, emotional, and physical well-being. While some people may effectively manage trauma in their youth, others may suffer its consequences later in life. Trauma in the latter stages of life can present distinct challenges and complications.

The growing global population of elderly individuals, expected to reach 1.2 billion by 2025, highlights the importance of addressing trauma among aging populations. Cumulative trauma, resulting from multiple traumatic experiences over a lifetime, becomes more prevalent with age and increases the risk of poor psychiatric outcomes, including PTSD. Elderly individuals are vulnerable to various sources of trauma, including maltreatment and abuse, both at home and in institutional settings like nursing homes. Acts of abuse, ranging from physical restraint to emotional neglect, can have severe and long-lasting psychological consequences, such as depression and anxiety.

Data on elder maltreatment is limited but suggests alarming rates of abuse, with a significant proportion of nursing home staff admitting to witnessing or committing acts of abuse. Social isolation, experienced by both caregivers and older adults, contributes to the risk of elder maltreatment and underscores the need for support services for both parties.

In addition to interpersonal trauma, older adults are susceptible to community traumas, such as natural disasters or terrorist attacks, and individual micro-traumas, like coping with a spouse's Alzheimer's diagnosis. These experiences can lead to feelings of "ambiguous loss" or "disenfranchised grief," particularly among marginalized groups within the elderly population.

It's crucial to recognize that the nature of trauma among older adults varies across ethnic and racial groups, highlighting the importance of culturally sensitive approaches to trauma intervention and support services. Addressing trauma among aging populations requires comprehensive strategies that prioritize prevention, early intervention, and support for both survivors and caregivers (Straussner & Calnan, 2014).

Types of Trauma Seniors May Experience

Trauma in seniors can manifest in various forms, stemming from a range of adverse experiences encountered throughout their lives. Here are some common types of trauma that seniors may experience.

Interpersonal Trauma

This includes physical, emotional, or sexual abuse, neglect, or exploitation by caregivers, family members, or others in positions of authority. Elder abuse can occur at home, in nursing homes, or in other care institutions.

Historical Trauma

Seniors may have suffered trauma from historical events such as war, violence, genocide, or forced displacement. These encounters have the potential to impact mental health and well-being across generations.

Medical Trauma

Seniors may have been exposed to stressful medical experiences such as surgery, hospitalizations, chronic illnesses, or serious health diagnoses. Invasive treatments, complications, or painful and distressing encounters can all cause medical trauma.

Loss and Bereavement

Seniors may face substantial losses, such as the death of spouses, partners, friends, or family members, as well as the loss of independence, mobility, or cognitive function. Grief can cause profound trauma and suffering.

Natural Disasters

Seniors may have been traumatized by natural disasters like hurricanes, earthquakes, floods, or wildfires. These disasters can result in property loss, displacement, disruption of community networks, and feelings of dread and vulnerability.

Community Violence

Seniors living in high-crime neighborhoods or areas with social unrest may experience trauma related to community violence, including witnessing a crime, gang activity, or civil chaos. Exposure to violence can contribute to feelings of insecurity and distress.

Discrimination and Marginalization

Seniors from marginalized or minority groups may have experienced trauma related to discrimination, prejudice, or social exclusion based on factors such as race, ethnicity, gender, sexual orientation, or socioeconomic status. Systemic oppression and injustice can have long-term effects on mental health and well-being.

Financial Exploitation

Seniors may experience trauma due to financial exploitation, scams, fraud, or theft perpetrated by family members, caregivers, or strangers. Financial abuse can lead to feelings of betrayal, loss of trust, and financial insecurity.

Isolation and Loneliness

Seniors who are socially isolated or lonely may experience trauma caused by feelings of abandonment, neglect, or a lack of connection with others. Social isolation can lead to sadness, anxiety, and a deterioration in physical health.

Recognizing the broad spectrum of traumas that elders may have encountered is critical to delivering trauma-informed care and support (Atinga et al., 2018)(Quinn, 2023).

Recognizing Trauma Symptoms

Understanding trauma symptoms is essential for assisting people who have been through difficult events. These symptoms can manifest differently for each individual: It all depends on what happened, how severe it was, and how each individual handled it. Also, if a person had mental health issues before the trauma, this can influence how they respond.

In times of uncertainty and change, it is vital to check in on those we care about because the key to assisting others through a difficult time is understanding what is going on and being there for them. Recognizing trauma entails recognizing the many signs and symptoms that individuals can exhibit in response to experiencing or witnessing a painful or traumatic incident.

Emotional Symptoms

- feeling really scared or anxious

- being very sad or down

- feeling guilty or ashamed

- getting easily irritated or angry

- feeling numb or disconnected from emotions

- finding it hard to feel happy or enjoy things

Physical Symptoms

- trouble sleeping or sleeping too much

- feeling tired all the time

- muscle tension or body aches

- headaches or stomachaches

- not wanting to eat or eating too much

Behavioral Symptoms

- avoiding places or people that remind you of the trauma

- feeling on edge all the time, like something terrible might happen

- having trouble concentrating or making decisions

- using alcohol or drugs more than usual to cope

- pulling away from friends or family

- acting out in aggressive or risky ways

Cognitive Symptoms

- having scary thoughts or memories of the trauma pop into your head

- having nightmares or flashbacks about what happened

- finding it hard to focus or remember things

- thinking negatively about yourself or the world

- feeling like things aren't natural or normal

Relational Symptoms

- having a hard time getting along with family, friends, or coworkers

- finding it tough to trust others or make new friends

- keeping to yourself and avoiding social situations

- relying too much on others for support

- having arguments or not communicating well with people

Many of those symptoms could be mistaken for something else, right? So, without knowing a person's specific experience, it may be challenging to determine whether these symptoms are a response to trauma. Remember, not everyone will exhibit all of these symptoms, which may vary over time. If you or someone you love is struggling due to a traumatic situation, you should get help from a professional (Nothaft, 2023; lyra Team, 2023).

The Role of Somatic Therapy in Trauma Healing

Somatic therapy is essential in trauma healing because it focuses on the relationship between the body and the mind. Trauma can have a profound influence on both physical and mental well-being, and somatic therapy helps people release stored trauma from their bodies. The primary purpose of somatic trauma therapy is to teach people how to become aware of these physical changes through concentration and mindfulness. They become aware of their body's reactions to emotional experiences, such as those caused by traumatic or highly stressful situations.

The trauma response is a natural reaction to extreme stress or life-threatening situations, where the brain and body quickly perceive danger and react to ensure survival. This response involves increased blood pressure and heart rate, heightened focus, and suppression of nonessential bodily functions like digestion. Known as the flight, fight, or freeze response, it prompts individuals to flee, fight, or immobilize in the face of danger. While the body usually returns to its normal state after the threat passes, in cases of continued perceived threat, stress responses persist, leading to conditions like PTSD and related physical and mental symptoms.

Somatic experience is a therapy that focuses on how the body responds to trauma and aids in healing. It is founded on an awareness of our bodies' spontaneous reactions to stressful events, such as feeling frozen or distant. This therapy aims to reduce bodily and emotional suffering by releasing grasped energy from these responses.

Somatic experiencing involves working with a therapist to become more aware of bodily sensations and feel more present in your body. This includes gentle techniques such as tapping or labeling body components. The therapist assists you in creating a safe environment to manage any overpowering feelings that may develop during therapy.

Then, using a technique known as titration, you progressively return to painful memories or feelings to digest them without being overwhelmed. Your therapist will walk you through this process, helping you recognize physical or emotional changes and allowing for emotional releases like crying or shaking. After that, you're directed back to a more relaxed condition called pendulation.

Overall, somatic therapy is essential in trauma recovery because it acknowledges the body's inherent wisdom and promotes internal healing. By addressing the somatic effects of trauma, individuals can experience profound shifts in their well-being and begin a journey toward healing and recovery (Porteous & Sebouhian, 2022)(Porrey, 2024).

Chapter 4: Somatic Approaches to Stress Reduction

A somatic approach involves directly concentrating our attention on the body's current feeling of anxiety and drawing on our own resources—breath, sensation, movement, and touch—to assist regulate the nervous system and relax the musculature.

It involves stress reduction through strategies that focus on the body's bodily sensations and motions to reduce stress and increase relaxation. These techniques emphasize the complex relationship between the mind and body, acknowledging that stress and trauma can appear both physically and cognitively.

Individuals can learn to regulate their nervous system, release tension, and nurture a sense of serenity and well-being by engaging in stress-reduction activities and practices. Somatic techniques include deep breathing exercises, progressive muscle relaxation, yoga, tai chi, massage therapy, and mindfulness meditation. Individuals can improve their self-awareness, resilience, and stress management skills using these approaches.

Mind-Body Connection

The mind-body connection refers to how your thoughts are linked to your emotions. The term "feelings" refers to physical sensations perceived in the body. The way someone thinks influences how they feel, and vice versa. So, according to this theory, negative ideas affect both the mind and the body. This concept of the mind-body connection opens up a therapeutic pathway for trauma, stress, anxiety, addiction, and other mental health illnesses (Quinn, 2023a).

The mind-body connection is the constant communication between our brain and body, involving the spinal cord, neurotransmitters, and hormones. It's responsible for processing information from our senses and sending signals for action throughout the body. An example of this connection is the fight-flight-or-freeze response, triggered when we sense danger. This response involves the sympathetic nervous system (gas pedal) preparing the body for action and the parasympathetic nervous system (brakes) calming it down afterward.

Somatization, or the physical expression of emotions and stress through the mind-body connection, is common and natural. It can occur independently, intensify existing medical conditions, or arise from distress caused by illness. For instance, a teenager experiencing fainting episodes due to stress, worsening gastrointestinal symptoms during periods of anxiety, or recurring headaches following a resolved concussion exemplifies somatization. Recognizing and understanding the mind-body connection can help manage physical symptoms related to emotions and stress.

Somatic therapy recognizes that psychological disorders

frequently show as physical symptoms and vice versa, highlighting the significance of incorporating bodily experiences into the therapeutic process. Somatic therapists work with people to investigate and comprehend how emotional stress, trauma, and unconscious patterns are stored in the body. Individuals learn to relax, process emotions, and restore balance to the mind-body system by using practices like body awareness, movement, touch, and breathwork (Vogels, 2019; Ra McComas, 2023).

Breathwork and Relaxation Techniques

Breathwork and relaxation techniques are essential components of somatic therapy, as they focus on utilizing the power of the breath to induce relaxation, reduce stress, and encourage emotional release. These treatments frequently include focused breathing exercises, guided imagery, progressive muscle relaxation, and meditation activities designed to soothe the nervous system and foster inner peace. Individuals can manage their physiological responses, calm the mind, and access deeper layers of awareness by focusing on the breath and encouraging deep, diaphragmatic breathing. Individuals who practice regularly can develop better stress resilience, cultivate a deeper connection to their bodies, and unlock the potential for profound healing and transformation.

Breathwork involves techniques that require conscious control of inhaling, exhaling, and breath retention, sometimes combined with specific movements or visualizations. This practice can help reduce stress, increase relaxation, improve focus, release tension, and facilitate emotional processing. It is used in various therapeutic contexts, including somatic therapy, mindfulness practices, and stress management interventions, offering a powerful tool for promoting holistic health and healing.

Relaxation approaches frequently involve consciously slowing down the body and mind, resulting in a relaxation reaction that counteracts the body's stress response. Common relaxation techniques include deep breathing exercises, gradual muscle relaxation, guided imagery, meditation, mindfulness, and visualization. These activities can be done alone or in combination, and they are commonly employed in various situations, including therapy, wellness programs, and self-care routines. Some of the breathwork and relaxation techniques are explained below.

Ideas for Getting Started

Breathing exercises do not have to be time-consuming. Set aside time to focus on your breathing. Here are a few ideas for getting started:

- Begin with simply five minutes every day and gradually increase the time as the exercise gets easier and more comfortable.
- If five minutes seems too long, start with two minutes.
- Practice several times per day. Schedule specific periods or practice aware breathing whenever you feel the urge.

Biodynamic Breathwork

Biodynamic breathwork is a six-element trauma release technique that combines breath, movement, music, touch, emotions, and meditation. This breathwork-to-heal trauma technique focuses on empowering your body, relieving tension, and reconstructing inner systems at the cellular level. Trauma causes fight-or-flight responses. The muscles and neurological system then store these responses. To assist with coping and processing, biodynamic breathwork provides a trauma-release approach that focuses on eliminating these blocks. Biodynamic breathwork and trauma release blend breathing with the intuitive downward and upward movements of your spine. This technique helps trauma and depression, improves focus and attention-deficit disorders, improves emotional integration, and encourages spiritual connection and aliveness.

Part 1

Stand with your feet shoulder-width apart and gently bend your knees.

1. Close your eyes and tune into your body.

2. Begin breathing in and out through your mouth without pausing.

3. As you breathe, move your head, face, and jaw intuitively in a patternless motion.

4. After some rounds of breath, begin intuitively moving your arms and shoulders.

5. Continue moving without pattern, allowing movement to radiate through you like a snake.

6. Keeping the energy moving downwards, start moving through your pelvis and unwinding your body.

7. Notice any trembling, tingling, or sensations and allow them to move through you.

8. Continue breathing and moving.

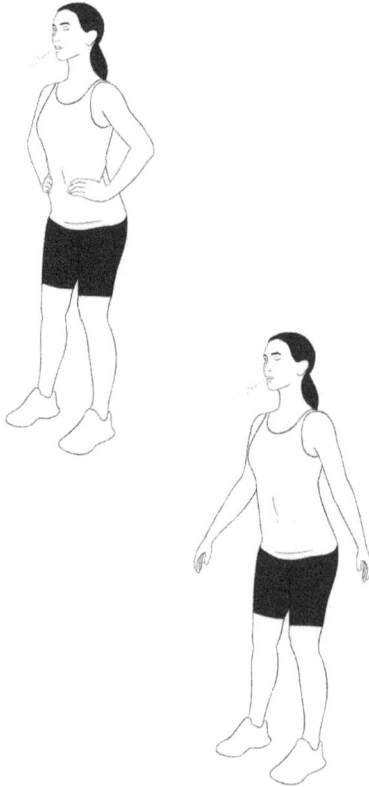

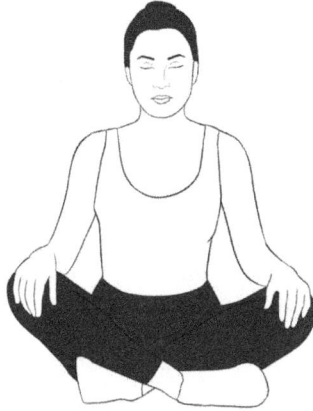

Part 2

Sit down on a mat or comfortable floor with your legs crossed and spine erect.

1. Change the direction of your movement upwards, moving from your core.

2. Breathe in and out, taking as many rounds of breath as feel good.

Part 3

When you're ready, lay down on your side with your knees bent and your hand under your head.

1. Breathe in and out.

2. Imagine movement radiating through you from the inside out.

3. Open your body by stretching your limbs and keep a flowing and unwinding movement as it feels good.

4. Lay on your back and move your pelvis.

5. Come into stillness when you feel ready.

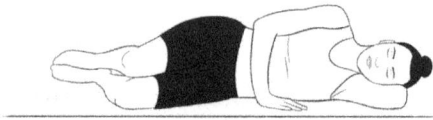

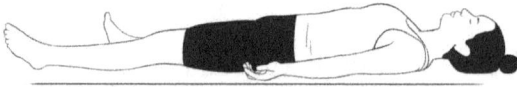

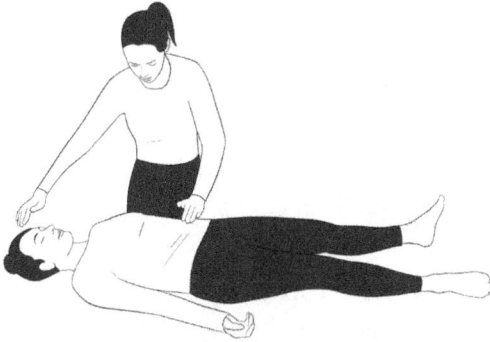

Holotropic Breathwork

This technique helps reach higher levels of self-awareness, alleviate depression, treat post-traumatic stress disorder, and combat addiction. Holotropic breathwork is derived from the Greek words holos (whole) and trepein (moving towards). This breathwork technique combines rapid breathing with emotive music while lying down. Holotropic breathing takes the practitioner into a non-ordinary level of consciousness, which is supposed to initiate a natural healing process and link you with your inner intellect.

1. Holotropic breathwork is often led by a facilitator, online or in-person, while evocative music plays in the background.

2. Lay down comfortably, eyes closed, or wearing an eye mask.

3. Breathe in and out via your lips, taking full breaths with no gap between them.

4. Keep breathing intuitively while listening to music.

5. Allow any emotions or sensations to express themselves

through music or movement—this is how you connect with your inner wisdom.

6. The holotropic breathwork facilitator will take you back into a state of relaxation.

The Wim Hof Method

The Wim Hof Method focuses on managing the autonomic nervous system to keep us from being pushed beyond our tolerance threshold. It works by inducing deep, oxygen-rich breaths that alter our heart rate variability. This breathing technique may also include intentional exposure to cold, which prevents our sympathetic system from activating and improves our ability to handle stress.

1. Sit or lie down comfortably, eyes closed.

2. Breathe in through the nose and out through the mouth completely, extending your belly on the inhales.

3. Repeat 30–40 breaths with short, forceful blasts of air. Lightheadedness and tingling are usual sensations here.

4. Finish your last exhale and inhale deeply for one more breath. Hold your breath for as long as possible. Then, take a large inhale with an expanded chest and belly. Hold for 15 seconds, then let go.

5. Repeat this breath cycle 3–4 times without pausing.

6. Repeat as needed.

Tips

- You can begin practicing most of these breath exercises right now. Take the opportunity to experiment with various breathing techniques.

- Set aside a specific amount of time at least a couple of times a week. You can repeat these workouts throughout the day.

- If you feel uncomfortable or dizzy, breathe naturally and get medical attention if necessary.

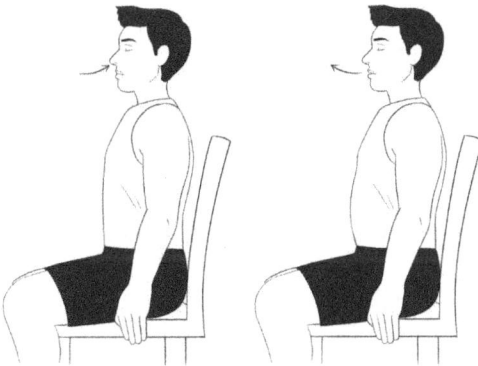

Progressive Muscle Relaxation

Progressive muscular relaxation is a two-step procedure that involves systematically tensing and relaxing various muscle groups in the body. With continuous practice, you will become intimately aware of the sensations of tension and perfect relaxation in multiple places of your body. This might help you respond to the initial signals of muscular tension that come with stress. And when your body relaxes, so does your mind.

Progressive muscular relaxation can be used with deep breathing to reduce stress. Consult your doctor first if you have a history of muscular spasms, back issues, or other significant ailments that tensing muscles could exacerbate. Begin at your feet and work your way up to your face, tensing only the muscles you desire.

1. Loosen your clothes, remove your shoes, and become comfortable.

2. Spend a few minutes inhaling and exhaling slowly and deeply.

3. When you're ready, focus your attention on your right foot. Take time to concentrate on how it feels.

4. Slowly tension the muscles in your right foot, squeezing as tightly as possible. Hold for a count of 10.

5. Relax your foot. Concentrate on releasing tension as well as the sensation of your foot going limp and loose.

6. Hold this relaxed posture for a moment, breathing deeply and slowly.

7. Direct your attention to your left foot. Follow the same muscle tension and release sequence.

8. Move gently up your body, contracting and relaxing each muscle group.

9. It may take some practice at first but try not to tighten muscles other than those needed.

Visualization

Visualization, often known as guided imagery, is a type of meditation in which you see yourself at peace, free of tension and anxiety. Choose a relaxing environment, such as a tropical beach, a childhood favorite, or a peaceful forested area. It will be used to reduce anxiety, and tension and enhance relaxation.

1. Close your eyes and envision yourself in a peaceful location.

2. Imagine everything you see, hear, smell, taste, and feel. Simply "looking" at it in your mind's eye, as if it were a snapshot, is insufficient.

3. Visualization works best when you include as many sensory elements as possible. For example, if you are considering a pier on a peaceful lake:

   ☐ Watch the sunset over the sea.

   ☐ Hear the birds sing.

   ☐ Smell the pine trees.

   ☐ Feel the chilly water against your naked feet.

   ☐ Taste the fresh, clear air.

4. Enjoy the sensation of your problems fading away as you leisurely explore your peaceful environment.

5. When you are ready, softly open your eyes and return to the present.

Stay calm if you occasionally zone out or lose track of where you are during a visualization session. This is normal. You may also notice heaviness in your limbs, muscle twitching, or yawning. Again, these are normal responses.

Self-Massage

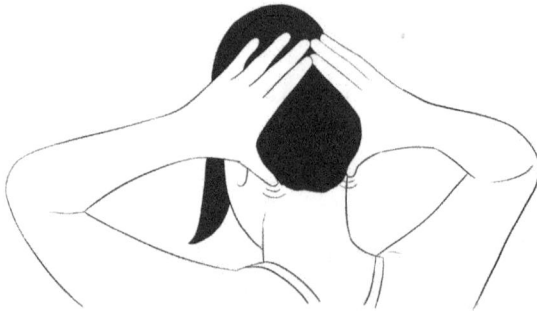

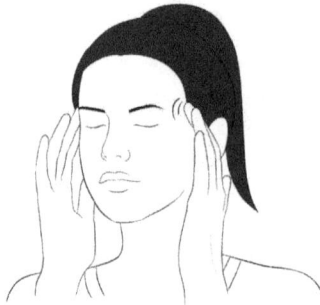

A combination of strokes effectively relieves muscle tightness. Try delicate chops with the edge of your hands, tapping with fingers, or cupped palms. Apply fingertip pressure to muscular knots. Kneel across muscles and try long, gentle, gliding strokes. You can use these strokes on any portion of your body that is conveniently accessible. For a short session, try focusing on your neck and head:

1. Begin by kneading the muscles at the back of your neck and shoulders. Make a loose fist and move it quickly up and down the sides and back of your neck. Next, use your thumbs to make little circles around the base of your skull. Gently massage the rest of your scalp with your fingertips. Then, touch your fingers against your scalp, going from front to back and over the sides.

2. Now, massage your face. Create a succession of little circles with your thumbs or fingertips. Pay close attention to your temples, forehead, and jaw muscles. Massage the bridge of your nose with your middle fingers, then work your way outward along your brows and temples.

3. Finally, close your eyes. Cup your hands loosely over your face and inhale and exhale efficiently for a short while.

Mindfulness Meditation

Mindfulness involves focusing on the current moment rather than lingering on the past or worrying about the future. It reduces tension, anxiety, and unpleasant emotions by increasing awareness and participation in present situations. This practice can include meditation, focusing on the breath or repetitive tasks, or incorporating mindfulness into daily activities. While learning may take time, the advantages include increased mental clarity and well-being. Using apps or audio tutorials can help novices acquire this practice.

1. Find a peaceful location where you will not be interrupted or distracted.

2. Sit in a comfy chair with your back straight.

3. Close your eyes and concentrate on something, such as your breathing—the sensation of air moving into and out of your nose or the rising and falling of your belly— or a meaningful word that you repeat throughout the meditation.

4. Do not worry about distracting ideas or how well you are doing. If thoughts interrupt your relaxation session, don't resist them; instead, softly return your attention to your area of focus without judgment.

Rhythmic Movement and Mindful Exercise

Exercising may not sound particularly soothing, but rhythmic exercise that gets you into a flow of repetitive movement can produce a relaxation response. Examples include

- running

- walking

- swimming

- dancing

- rowing

- climbing

For maximum stress relief, add mindfulness to your workout.

Tips

- Learning the fundamentals of these relaxation techniques is simple, but maximizing their stress-relieving potential requires consistent practice.

- Try to set aside 10 to 20 minutes per day for your relaxation practice.

- Set aside some time in your everyday agenda. If feasible, schedule your practice time once or twice a day.

Integrating Breathwork With Movement

Integrating breathwork with movement includes matching your breathing patterns with various physical activities to improve mindfulness and overall well-being. One method is to sync your breath with the rhythm of your movements, such as inhaling during one phase and exhaling during another. For example, in yoga, you might inhale as you raise your arms aloft and exhale as you fold forward. Another technique is to focus on deep, diaphragmatic breathing while walking, stretching, or dancing, which can assist in relaxing the mind and promote bodily awareness. Remember to keep a steady and relaxed breathing rhythm throughout the motions. Some of the techniques are explained below.

Diaphragmatic Breathing

Practice diaphragmatic breathing for 5–10 minutes, 3 to 4 times daily. When you begin, you may feel tired, but the technique should become easier and more natural over time. This technique is used to support healing, have higher energy levels, and experience better mental or creative focus through specific breathing methods.

1. Lie on your back with your knees slightly bent and your head on a pillow.

2. You may place a pillow under your knees for support.

3. Place one hand on your upper chest and one hand below your rib cage, allowing you to feel the movement

of your diaphragm.

4. Slowly inhale through your nose, feeling your stomach pressing into your hand.

5. Keep your other hand as still as possible.

6. Exhale using pursed lips as you tighten your abdominal muscles, keeping your upper hand completely still.

You can place a book on your abdomen to make the exercise more challenging. Once you learn how to do belly breathing lying down, you can increase the difficulty by trying it while sitting in a chair. You can then practice the technique while performing your daily activities (Cronkleton, 2019).

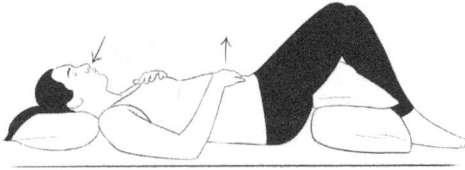

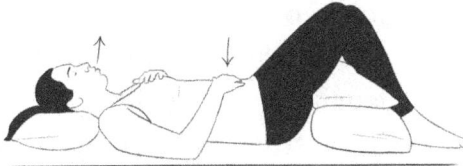

Laughter Yoga

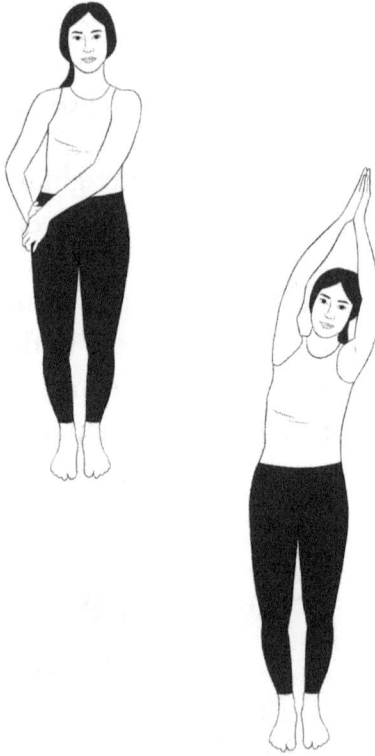

Madan Kataria popularized laughter yoga, which includes intentional, manufactured laughter, and has received widespread attention for its multiple health advantages. Research published in Current Research in Physiology discovered that laughter improves lung function and circulation and reduces stress levels by producing feel-good brain chemicals such as dopamine, oxytocin, endorphins, and serotonin. Because the brain cannot distinguish between genuine and synthetic laughter, both can deliver identical benefits, making laughter yoga a fun and effective form of breathwork practice. It is used to lower anxiety, boost self-esteem, increase happiness, relieve gastrointestinal problems, and possibly even lose weight.

You might simply start laughing, smiling, and applauding to get the advantages of this activity, but if you want a more structured approach, follow these steps.

1. Cross your right hand over to meet your left hand at your left hip and clap your hands while exhaling "ho ho." Do this from a confident standing position, smiling.

2. Pull the arms up on a diagonal to the right side of the head, clapping and exhaling "ha ha ha."

3. Repeat this three times. After the final "ha ha ha," raise both arms above your head and yell, "Yay!" before laughing.

Vinyasa Yoga

Vinyasa yoga is a dynamic and fluid type of yoga that combines movement and breathing. Vinyasa practice involves students moving through a series of positions in a flowing sequence, with each movement linked to an inhale or an exhale. The transitions between positions are seamless and consistent, resulting in a rhythmic flow. Vinyasa sessions vary in intensity and pace, giving options for both beginners and advanced practitioners. This yoga practice improves strength, flexibility, and balance and fosters mindfulness and relaxation by linking breath to movement.

1. Begin by standing comfortably, feet hip-width apart, hands by your sides.

2. Take a few deep breaths to center yourself and concentrate on your goal for the session.

3. Begin with a light warm-up, such as neck rolls, shoulder rolls, and stretches, to prepare your body for activity.

4. Form a series of positions, transitioning from one to the next with each inhale and exhale. Vinyasa yoga's most common poses are Downward Facing Dog, Plank Pose, Upward Facing Dog, and Child's Pose.

5. Coordinate your breathing with each movement, inhaling as you lift or extend and exhaling as you fold or release.

6. Pay attention to your posture and use your core muscles to support your movement.

7. Smoothly transition between positions, keeping a steady and even breath throughout the practice.

8. Continue to move through the postures at your own pace, listening to and honoring your body's demands.

9. Finish the practice with a few minutes of Savasana, where you lie on your back with your eyes closed and focus on your breathing.

10. When you're ready, gently return to a seated position and place your hands on your heart center, honoring the time and work you've put into your practice.

11. Remember to listen to your body and alter poses as needed to suit your specific degree of flexibility and strength.

Tips

To incorporate these breathwork techniques into your movement practice

- Begin by practicing them one at a time. As you become more comfortable with the techniques, you can incorporate them into your movement sessions before, after, or even during.

- Observe how they affect your energy levels and state of mind.

- Listen to your body and take breaks as needed.

Chapter 5: Mindful Movement Sequences

Sequences of physical exercises or activities known as mindful movement practices are carried out with conscious attention to the present moment and frequently include aspects of body awareness, breath awareness, and mindfulness. Depending on the particular practice or activity, these sequences might vary considerably. Still, they usually feature deliberate, slow motions to encourage relaxation, stress reduction, and an improved mind-body connection. A few sequences of conscious movements are as follows.

Mindful movement sequences involve flowing through a series of yoga or tai chi poses, with focused attention on the present moment.

Here's a Simple Mindful Movement Sequence

1. Begin in a comfortable standing position with your feet hip-width apart and arms relaxed by your sides. Take a few deep breaths to center yourself.

2. On an inhale, raise your arms overhead, reaching up towards the sky, and gently arch your back. Exhale as you return to the starting position.

3. Inhale and sweep your arms out to the sides, coming into a gentle twist to the right. Exhale as you return to the center, then repeat the twist to the left.

4. Lower your torso toward your legs and hinge at the hips to begin the forward fold. To maintain a long spine, bend your knees as much as necessary.

5. Take a deep breath, stretch your back, and plant your hands on your thighs or shins to begin the Halfway Lift. Then, push your chest forward.

6. Let go of any tightness in your shoulders and neck by exhaling as you fold forward again.

7. Lower your right knee to the mat by stepping your right foot back into a lunge. Breathe in as you enter the Low Lunge by sweeping your arms overhead. Breathe out as you put your hands back on the mat.

8. Return to Plank Pose by stepping your left foot back to meet your right. Hold while using your core muscles for a few breaths.

9. With control, lower yourself to the mat, and then inhale into Cobra Pose to gently come into a backbend. As you let go again, release a breath.

10. Return to Child's Pose, putting your arms out in front of you and placing your forehead on the mat. Take a few deep breaths to help your body unwind and release any tension.

11. When you're prepared, return to a seated position and observe your feelings following the process for a short while. Think back on any feelings or experiences you had during the exercise.

You can develop an awareness of your breath, body, and thoughts as you go through the poses in this mindful movement sequence by practicing purpose and presence. You can change the order to fit your tastes and skill level. Following are some examples of mindful movement sequences:

1. Yoga Flow

2. Tai Chi

3. Qigong

4. Pilates

5. Walking Meditation

6. Mindful Stretching

7. Functional Movement Patterns

8. Mindful Strength Training

Fluid Transitions Between Exercises

Fluid transitions between exercises, particularly in yoga or dance, entail smoothly transitioning from one posture or movement to the next without interruptions or abrupt changes. These transitions are important for preserving the rhythm and continuity of the practice, improving the overall experience, and lowering the chance of injury.

To attain this fluidity, practitioners highlight several critical components. To begin, they synchronize their motions with the breath, matching inhales and exhales with particular actions to create a smooth and rhythmic flow.

Furthermore, practitioners are fully present in each moment, allowing them to anticipate forthcoming movements and modify their bodies accordingly, ensuring balance, alignment, and focus throughout the transition. To achieve smooth transitions, practitioners rely on several key elements:

- **Breath awareness:**

  Coordinating motions with the breath promotes a smooth and rhythmic flow. Expansive or opening movements frequently accompany inhales whereas exhales are connected with contracting or grounded moves.

- **Mindfulness:**

  Being completely present in each moment enables practitioners to anticipate the following action and change their bodies accordingly. Mindfulness also assists in maintaining balance, alignment, and focus during the transition.

- **Alignment and stability:**

  Proper alignment and stability in each posture allow for a smooth transition to the next. Engaging core muscles and maintaining a steady base provide the framework for movement.

- **Transitional movements:**

  Incorporating transitional movements or poses between more complex workouts helps close the gap and smooths transitions. These movements might be simple and repetitive, acting as a bridge between other patterns.

- **Practice and awareness:**

  Regular practice and mindful awareness of movement

patterns will help you to master fluid transitions over time. Transitions become more effortless and natural as practitioners become more comfortable.

Here's How to Do It

A smooth transition between exercises in a mindful movement sequence could be from a standing forward fold (Uttanasana) to a low lunge (Anjaneyasana).

1. Begin by standing with feet hip-width apart and hands resting on your hips.

2. Inhale deeply to lengthen your spine and lift your chest.

3. As you exhale, hinge at the hips and gradually fold forward, bringing your hands to the floor or resting them on your shins or thighs.

4. On the next inhalation, raise halfway up, extending your spine and pulling your shoulder blades together.

5. Exhale and return your right foot to a lunge stance, stacking your left knee over your left ankle.

6. Lower your right knee softly to the ground and untuck your toes, placing the top of your right foot on the mat.

7. Inhale as you raise your arms aloft, falling into a low lunge with your body upright and your arms reaching for the sky.

8. Exhale and sink deeper into the lunge, allowing your hips to open and your chest to rise.

9. Hold the posture for a few breaths, paying attention to the sensations in your hips and thighs and the expansion of your chest with each inhalation.

10. To exit the posture, exhale and return your hands to the mat on each side of your left foot.

11. Step your left foot back to meet your right foot, then return to the forward fold posture.

12. Inhale and gradually roll up to standing, piling each vertebra on top of the next until you achieve a standing position.

13. Repeat the movement on the opposite side by stepping your left foot back into a lunge and elevating your right foot.

Seated, Standing, and Lying Down Exercises

Seated, standing, and lying down exercises are common types of movements used in fitness routines, yoga practices, physical therapy sessions, and mindfulness exercises. Each category focuses on distinct muscle areas and provides unique advantages.

Seated Exercises

Seated exercises are done while sitting in a chair or on the floor. They are helpful for people who have mobility problems, balance challenges, or prefer a low-impact workout. Seated exercises can work multiple muscle groups, such as the core, legs, arms, and back. Seated workouts include leg lifts, twists, forward folds, and arm movements using tension bands or weights.

Here are some examples!

Seated Forward Fold (Paschimottanasana)

- Sit on the floor, legs extended in front of you.

- Inhale to lengthen your spine, then exhale to hinge at the hips and fold forward, reaching for your toes.

- The hands are usually reaching towards the feet or ankles.

- Hold the stretch for several breaths, and feel the extending sensation throughout your spine and the back of your legs.

Benefits

- It massages pelvic and abdominal organs while toning the shoulders.

Seated Twist (Ardha Matsyendrasana)

- Sit cross-legged on the ground or in a chair.

- Inhale to stretch your spine, then exhale to twist to the right, with your left hand on your knee and your right hand behind you for support.

- Hold the twist for a few breaths before repeating on the opposing side.

Benefits

- It makes the spine more flexible.

- It increases the oxygen supply to the lungs.

Thunderbolt Pose (Vajrasana)

- Vajrasana is performed while sitting on the floor.

- Kneel on the floor and sit back on your heels, toes touching each other and knees splitting apart.

- The hands are put on the knees, while the back remains straight.

Benefits

- It is often performed after a meal to aid digestion and improve blood circulation.

- It is also said to help with stress and anxiety and strengthen the back and leg muscles.

Standing Exercises

Standing exercises are carried out while standing upright, with or without the assistance of a chair, wall, or other supports. These exercises work the muscles in the lower body, core, and stabilizers, which help improve balance, coordination, and general strength. Standing exercises frequently portray functional movements found in regular activity. Some examples are squats, lunges, calf raises, standing leg lifts, and yoga balance exercises such as tree position or warrior pose.

Here are some examples!

Sideways Bending Pose (Konasana)

- Konasana, commonly known as the Sideways Bending Pose, consists of reaching one arm towards the sky while standing.

- Rest the other arm upon the leg.

Benefits

- It helps increase flexibility, balance, and strength.

- It also helps in relieving stress and tension in the spine and hips.

- It also helps those suffering from constipation.

Chair Pose (Utkatasana)

- Utkatasana, also known as Chair Pose, is a strengthening yoga posture that works the legs, back, and core muscles.

- The knees are bent, and the hips are lowered as if sitting in an imaginary chair.

- Arms are raised overhead to complete the pose.

Benefits

- It strengthens the lower back and torso.

- It balances the body and promotes willpower.

Tree Pose (Vrksasana)

- Stand tall, feet hip-width apart.

- Transfer your weight to your left foot and lift your right foot off the ground.

- Place the sole of your right foot on your left inner thigh or calf, avoiding the knee.

- Bring your palms together at your heart's center or raise your arms overhead.

- Find a focus point to help with balance, then hold the pose for a few breaths before switching sides.

Benefits

- It increases focus.

- It makes the legs strong, improves balance, and opens the hip.

- It also helps those suffering from sciatica, a pain that travels from the pelvic region through the hips and thighs.

Lying Down Exercises

These exercises are done while lying on your back, stomach, or side. These exercises primarily target the core, back, hips, and leg muscles. Lying down exercises can enhance flexibility, mobility, and posture while putting less load on the joints. Examples include bridges, leg raises, crunches, planks, side-leg lifts, and supine twists.

Here are some examples:

Corpse Pose (Savasana)

- Lie on your back, legs extended, arms at your sides, palms up.

- Close your eyes and relax your entire body to relieve tension or stress.

- Concentrate on your breath and allow yourself to settle into the present moment.

- Remain in this pose for a few minutes to reap the advantages of deep relaxation.

Benefits

- It brings a deep, meditative state of rest.

- It helps reduce blood pressure, anxiety, and insomnia.

Supine Twist

- Lie on your back, arms stretched to the sides in a T-shape.

- Bend your knees and draw them up to your chest.

- Exhale and lower both knees to the right while maintaining your upper back and shoulders grounded.

- Turn your head to the left and look at your left hand. Hold the twist for a few breaths before repeating on the opposite side.

Benefits

- It brings deep relaxation to the body and mind.

- It strengthens the legs, improves balance and stability, and stretches the chest, back, and hip muscles.

Bridge Pose (Setu Bandhasana)

- Lie on your back, knees bent, feet hip-width apart.

- Lift your hips towards the ceiling by pressing onto your feet and using your glutes and thighs.

- Place your arms alongside your body, palms down.

- Push your upper arms down.

- Hold the pose for a few breaths to feel your chest's stretch and your legs' strength.

Benefits

- It helps calm the brain.

- It helps to reduce anxiety.

- It helps minimize thyroid problems (Pizer, 2013; Orenstein, 2019).

Personalization and Adaptations

Personalization

Personalization in exercise is the process of adapting workout programs to individual needs, goals, and abilities, considering variables such as fitness level, preferences, and health problems. This method maximizes effectiveness and safety by altering intensity, exercise selection, and addressing any existing health concerns or injuries. Personalized programs foster greater engagement and adherence, hence promoting long-term health and fitness goals. Here is a thorough overview:

- **Assessment:** Personalization begins with a comprehensive evaluation of the individual's fitness level, health status, medical history, exercise experience, and goals. This may include body composition, cardiovascular fitness, strength, flexibility, and mobility examinations. Understanding these elements helps to establish a baseline from which to build a personalized plan.

- **Goal setting:** Following the evaluation, specific, measurable, attainable, relevant, and time-bound (SMART) goals are developed in partnership with the individual. Such aims include weight loss, muscle building, increased endurance, flexibility, injury avoidance, and sports-specific performance objectives. Goals should be realistic and align with the individual's aspirations and motivations.

- **Customized exercise selection:** Personalization means selecting or adapting workouts corresponding to the individual's goals, interests, and talents. This could involve selecting exercises that target specific muscle groups, movement patterns, or fitness components related to the individual's goals. Exercise selection may vary depending on equipment availability, space limitations, and the individual's interests.

- **Intensity and progression:** The intensity and progression of exercises are tailored to each individual's fitness level, tolerance, and goals. This includes adjusting variables like resistance, repetitions, sets, tempo, rest periods, and exercise frequency to keep exercises tough but reasonable. Progression should be gradual, based on gains in strength, endurance, or other fitness metrics,

- **Individual preferences and enjoyment:** Personalization considers the individual's preferences, hobbies, and lifestyle circumstances to increase fitness program adherence and enjoyment. This could incorporate activities the individual enjoys, such as dance, swimming, hiking, or group fitness programs. Offering variety and opportunities for exploration encourages people to choose activities that are relevant to their interests and keeps them motivated to exercise regularly.

- **Feedback and monitoring:** Continuous feedback and monitoring are critical components of personalization to measure success, identify areas for growth, and provide inspiration and support. This can include regular check-ins, performance assessments, communication with a fitness professional or coach, and self-monitoring strategies like keeping a workout diary or using fitness tracking apps.

Adaptation

Adaptation in exercise refers to the physiological and functional changes due to frequent physical activity. When exposed to exercise stressors, the body adapts to become more efficient and resilient. These adaptations occur across multiple systems, including muscular, cardiovascular, metabolic, neuromuscular, and flexibility.

- **Stimulus and response:** When the body is subjected to exercise stressors such as resistance training, cardiovascular exercise, or flexibility training, it responds by causing physiological changes to match the demands of the activity. This stimulus causes a sequence of adaptive responses in the body.

- **Muscle adaptation:** Resistance training, such as weightlifting or bodyweight workouts, causes microtears in muscle fibers, leading to muscular adaptation. In reaction, the body heals and strengthens these fibers, resulting in muscle growth (hypertrophy) and enhanced strength. Over time, the muscles adapt to the stress of exercise.

- **Cardiovascular adaptation:** Cardiovascular exercise, such as running, cycling, or swimming, causes changes in the cardiovascular system. This includes improved heart function, such as increased stroke volume (the quantity of blood pumped with each heartbeat) and cardiac output (the volume of blood pumped per minute), as well as increased blood supply to working muscles and better oxygen delivery efficiency.

- **Metabolic adaptation:** Exercise induces metabolic changes that improve energy production and utilization. Regular physical exercise enhances the body's ability to use oxygen (aerobic capacity), increases mitochondrial density (the energy-producing organelles inside cells), improves insulin sensitivity, and boosts fat oxidation. These adaptations help to boost endurance, energy, and metabolic health.

- **Neuromuscular adaptation:** Exercise also triggers neuromuscular adaptations, which include the nervous system's control over muscle function. This has enhanced motor unit recruitment, coordination, balance, proprioception (awareness of body location), and muscle activation patterns. These adjustments help to improve movement efficiency, production of power, and motor abilities.

- **Flexibility and mobility adaptation:** Stretching and mobility exercises generate muscle adaptations, tendon, ligament, and joint adaptations. Stretching regularly promotes muscle suppleness and joint range of motion, lowers muscular tension, and improves general flexibility and joint mobility. These changes enhance the quality of movement, reduce the chance of injury, and promote optimal biomechanics.

- **Individual variability:** Individuals' adaptation to exercise varies depending on genetics, age, gender, training history, nutrition, sleep, and lifestyle factors. Some people may have faster or more pronounced adaptations than others, while others may need more time or other training methods to obtain equal outcomes.

- **Progressive overload:** To continue to see adaptations and improvements in fitness, gradually increase the intensity, duration, or frequency of exercise over time. This idea of progressive overload ensures that the body is constantly challenged and stimulated to adapt to increased demands, resulting in continuous gains in strength, endurance, flexibility, and general fitness.

Understanding exercise adaptation enables individuals to create effective workout programs, set realistic goals, and optimize training tactics to enhance performance, avoid plateaus, and obtain long-term fitness and health advantages (Lambert, 2016; Hughes et al., 2017).

Chapter 6: Practical Somatic Exercises for Seniors

Implementing practical somatic exercises for elders is a gentle and effective technique to increase mobility, flexibility, and overall health. These exercises increase body awareness and relieve stress through mindful movement. One such exercise is the gentle neck roll, in which seniors carefully tilt their heads to one side, feeling the stretch throughout their neck and shoulder, and then repeat on the other side. This reduces stiffness and promotes relaxation.

Another useful exercise is the sitting spinal twist, which allows seniors to sit comfortably and slowly rotate their upper body from side to side, stretching the spine and increasing torso mobility. Seniors can practice the tree pose variation to improve their balance and stability by standing next to a sturdy chair, lifting one leg, and placing the foot on the inner thigh or calf of the standing leg. This pose strengthens the leg muscles and improves proprioception, essential for avoiding falls. Furthermore, seated leg lifts can assist seniors in developing their quadriceps and enhance lower body strength while sitting in a chair by elevating one leg at a time and holding for a few seconds before lowering it again.

Breathing exercises are also important components of somatic practices for elders, as they promote relaxation and reduce tension. One such practice is diaphragmatic breathing, in which elders can sit comfortably with their eyes closed and concentrate on breathing deeply into their abdomen, allowing it to rise on the inhale and fall on the exhale. This relaxes the nervous system and promotes a sense of inner serenity and well-being.

Overall, practical somatic exercises for elders provide moderate but effective methods for improving mobility, balance, and overall physical and mental health. Seniors who incorporate these activities into their routine can experience more vitality, less pain and stiffness, and better resilience in negotiating the obstacles of aging.

Diverse Range of Exercises

Somatic exercises for seniors include various motions to increase body awareness, flexibility, and overall well-being. These exercises are tailored to older persons' specific requirements and skills, providing light yet effective strategies to maintain physical and mental health. These exercises include gentle stretching, joint mobilization, balance training, mindful breathing practices, and mind-body integration. Somatic exercises can help seniors improve their physical performance, reduce pain, relax more, and have a better overall quality of life. Some of them are listed below.

Calming Breathing Technique

You can practice standing, sitting in a back-supporting chair, or reclining on a bed or yoga mat on the floor. Make yourself as comfortable as possible. If possible, loosen any clothing that is restricting your breathing. This technique is used to calm the nervous system that controls the body's involuntary functions, lower blood pressure and heart rate, and reduce stress hormone levels in the blood.

1. If you're lying down, position your arms slightly away from your sides, palms up. Keep your legs straight or bend your knees so your feet are flat on the ground.

2. If you are sitting, rest your arms on the chair arms.

3. Keep both feet flat on the floor if you're seated or standing. Place your feet about hip-width apart, regardless of your position.

4. Allow your breath to flow as deeply into your abdomen as is comfortable without forcing it.

5. Try inhaling through your nose and exhaling through your mouth.

6. Inhale slowly and regularly. Some people find it beneficial to count consistently from one to five. You may need help to reach five at first.

7. Allow it to flow out softly, counting from one to five again if necessary.

8. Repeat this for at least five minutes.

Breathing While In Pain

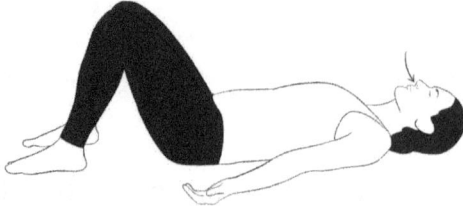

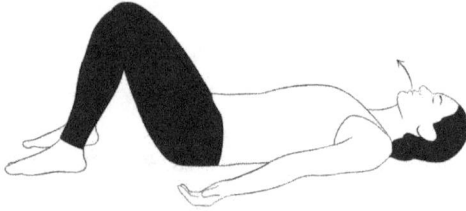

It is tough to breathe properly when in pain. This is because our bodies believe that holding our breath allows us to reduce pain and suffering. However, this exacerbates the pain by activating our stress reaction. Here's the appropriate method to breathe while in pain. The goal of breath-in-pain exercises is to employ focused breathing techniques to relieve physical discomfort and induce relaxation, allowing people to manage and cope with pain more successfully.

1. Get into a comfortable position in a quiet area.

2. Inhale as deeply and slowly as possible.

3. Fill your abdomen with air while your head remains relaxed and focused.

4. Slowly exhale to clear your airway.

5. Repeat the practice until breathing is more controlled.

Chinese Breathing

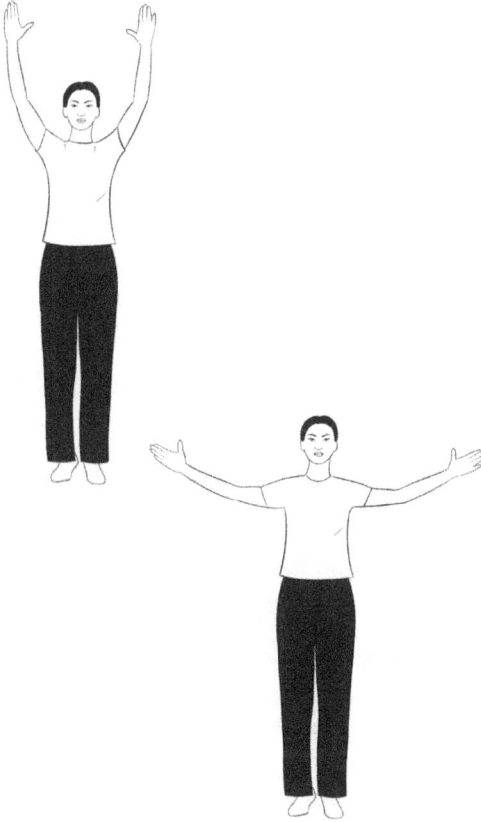

The exercise is based on the Chinese tradition of Tai Chi Chuan. This practice aims to cultivate a state of relaxation, enhance energy circulation, and support overall well-being.

1. Take three short breaths.

2. On the first breath, raise your arms to shoulder height in front of you.

3. Bring your arms up to shoulder height at your sides on your second breath.

4. Raise them above your head with your final breath.

5. Then, breathe softly and lower your arms back to your sides.

6. Try 10 to 12 repetitions. Stop exercising if you feel lightheaded.

Neck Rolls

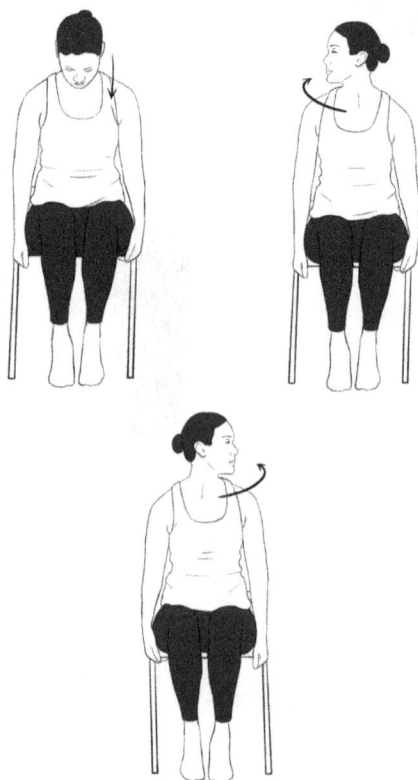

Neck rolls are a simple approach to relieve pain and improve your range of motion. Neck rolls and other stretches help you enhance your range of motion. Improving your neck's range of motion is essential for preventing pain caused by bad posture.

1. Sit comfortably on a chair, and maintain your posture in an erect position.

2. Start with your head down.

3. Roll around to the right.

4. Roll around to the back.

5. Roll around to the left.

6. Roll back down to the front.

7. Repeat three times (to the right).

8. Then, complete one set of 3 neck rolls to the left.

Seated Resistance Band Exercises

Seated resistance band exercises are simple yet effective workouts that can be done while sitting down, making them accessible for seniors or those with limited mobility. These seated resistance band exercises can help improve strength, flexibility, and mobility in the upper and lower body, all from the comfort of a chair.

1. Sit on a sturdy chair with a straight back and your feet flat on the floor.

2. Secure one end of the resistance band under your foot and hold the other end with your hand.

3. Start with a basic exercise like bicep curls. Hold the band with your palm facing upward, bend your elbow, and lift your hand toward your shoulder.

4. Perform 10–15 repetitions of the bicep curl, then switch to the other arm.

5. You can also do shoulder presses. Hold the band with your palms facing downward at shoulder height, then push upward until your arms are fully extended.

6. Again, do 10–15 repetitions of shoulder presses.

7. Secure the band around both feet and hold the ends with your hands for leg exercises.

8. Perform leg extensions by straightening one leg out in front of you against the resistance of the band, then return to the starting position.

9. Do 10–15 repetitions for each leg.

10. Remember to breathe steadily throughout the exercises and maintain good posture.

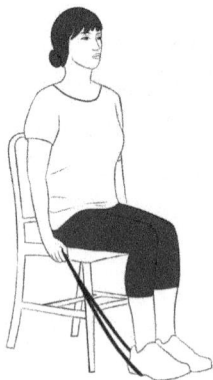

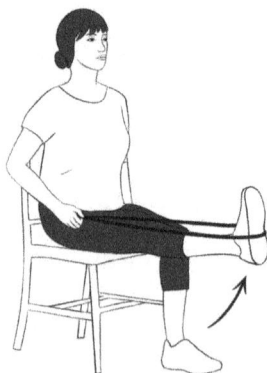

Qigong

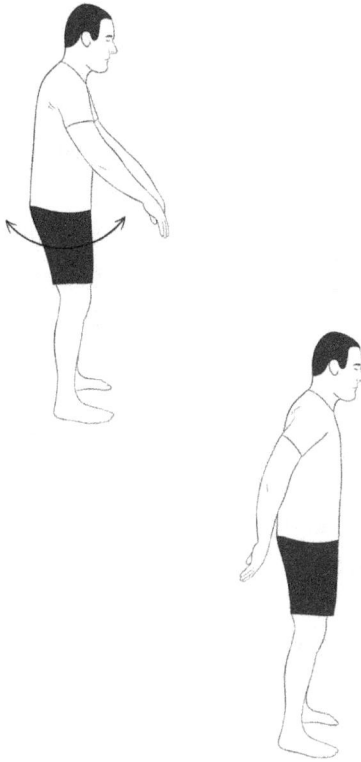

Qigong is a traditional Chinese practice that combines gentle movements, breath control, and meditation to promote health and well-being. This technique promotes harmony between the body, mind, and spirit, helping to enhance vitality, reduce stress, and improve overall health.

1. Begin by finding a comfortable standing or sitting position, ensuring your body is relaxed, and your feet are firmly planted on the ground.

2. Focus on your breath, taking slow, deep breaths through your nose and mouth. Imagine the breath

flowing smoothly through your body, filling you with energy and relaxation.

3. Start with gentle movements, such as swaying from side to side or raising and lowering your arms. Let the movements flow naturally with your breath, feeling the energy circulating through your body.

4. Stay present in the moment, paying attention to the sensations in your body and the rhythm of your breath. Let go of any distracting thoughts and focus on the here and now.

5. Set an intention for your practice, whether cultivating peace, reducing stress, or improving your health. Visualize yourself achieving your goal as you continue with the movements.

6. Repeat the movements for several minutes or longer, allowing yourself to sink deeper into relaxation with each breath. You can gradually increase the intensity or duration of your practice as you become more comfortable.

7. When you're ready to end your practice, take a few moments to return to stillness, allowing your body and mind to integrate the benefits of your Qigong session. Thank yourself for taking the time to nurture your well-being.

Body Scan Meditation

This meditation directs your attention to different parts of your body. Like gradual muscle relaxation, you begin with your feet and work your way up. Instead of tensing and releasing muscles, you concentrate on how each part of your body feels without categorizing the sensations as "good" or "bad." This technique examines your body for pain, stress, or anything out of the ordinary. It helps you feel more connected to your physical and emotional selves.

1. Lie on your back with your legs uncrossed, arms loose at your sides, and eyes open or closed. Concentrate on your breathing for around two minutes until you begin to feel relaxed.

2. Focus on the toes of your right foot. Take note of any sensations you experience while remaining focused on your breathing. Imagine each deep breath traveling to your toes. Stay focused on this area for three to five seconds.

3. Direct your attention to the sole of your right foot. Pay attention to any feelings you feel in that portion of your body, and envision each breath coming from the sole of your foot.

4. After a minute or two, shift your concentration to your right ankle and repeat.

5. Move to your calf, knee, thigh, and hip, then repeat for your left leg.

6. From there, go up the body, passing through the lower back and belly, the upper back and chest, and the

shoulders. Pay close attention to any part of your body that hurts or makes you uncomfortable.

7. After you've completed the body scan, sit quietly and still for a moment, taking note of how your body feels. Then, carefully open your eyes and stretch, if necessary.

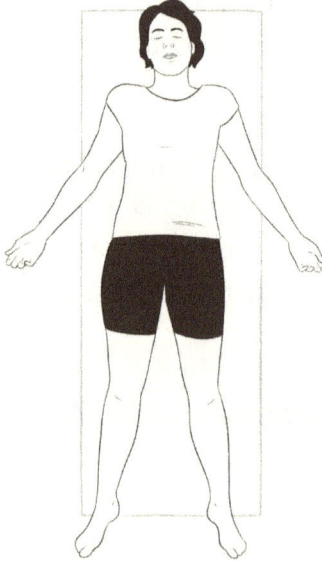

Interactive Elements

Interactive elements in senior exercise programs are essential for increasing engagement, motivation, and enjoyment, which leads to higher adherence and general well-being. Some interactive components that can be used in senior activities include:

- Gamification: Adding game-like features to workouts, such as challenges, rewards, and progress tracking, can increase engagement and enjoyment. Seniors, for example, might earn points or badges for doing specific exercises or meeting fitness milestones, which gives them a sense of success and encouragement.

- Technology integration: Using fitness applications, wearable devices, or virtual reality platforms, seniors can use interactive tools for tracking their progress, receiving feedback, and accessing guided workouts. These technologies can also provide individualized advice and tailor exercises to particular skills and goals.

- Social connection: Group exercises or team-based activities promote social connection and camaraderie among elders, providing a sense of belonging and support. Seniors can engage with others while participating in group exercises such as partner workouts, group walks, or team sports. Group exercises or team-based activities promote social connection and camaraderie among elders, providing a sense of belonging and support. Seniors can engage with others while participating in group exercises such as partner workouts, group walks, or team sports.

- Multi-sensory experiences: Engaging many senses, such

as sight, hearing, and touch, can make activities more participatory for seniors. For example, incorporating music, vibrant sights, or tactile objects into workouts can boost sensory perception and enhance the immersive and joyful experience.

- Mind-body connection: Incorporating mindfulness practices, relaxation techniques, or breathwork into activities helps seniors connect with their bodies and become more aware of physical sensations and emotions. Mind-body exercises encourage relaxation, stress reduction, and overall well-being, improving the training experience's interactive aspect. Incorporating mindfulness practices, relaxation techniques, or breathwork into activities helps seniors connect with their bodies and become more aware of physical sensations and emotions. Mind-body exercises encourage relaxation, stress reduction, and overall well-being, improving the training experience's interactive aspect.

Variety and Creativity

Providing various exercises and activities keeps elders engaged and minimizes boredom. Incorporating creative elements into workouts, such as dancing, art, or storytelling, adds variety and enjoyment, enabling seniors to remain active and interested in their exercise routine.

By incorporating interactive elements into exercises for seniors, whether through gamification, technology integration, social interaction, multi-sensory experiences, mind-body connection, or creative variety, fitness programs can be made more engaging, motivating, and enjoyable for older adults, promoting long-term adherence and improved overall health and well-being.

Here are some QR codes and resources. You can scan through them to get an idea of the interactive elements.

Top 5 Interactive Fitness Equipment for Adults

Interactive Fitness and Sport Equipment

10 interactive activities to stimulate the elderly at home

The Benefits of Using Interactive Fitness Equipment

Progressive Exercises for Strength and Flexibility

Progressive exercises for strength and flexibility involve gradually increasing the intensity or difficulty of movements over time. This helps improve muscle strength, endurance, and flexibility. Strength exercises are any activities that require the muscles to work harder than usual. They entail using body weight or working against resistance to enhance muscle strength, power, size, and endurance. Strength exercises should be demanding but not stressful. You should lift a weight that you can comfortably handle in multiple repetitions.

Flexibility exercises are activities that increase your joints' capacity to maintain the movement required for daily chores and physical activity. Flexibility refers to the range of motion in a joint or group of joints and the ability to move joints effectively across a full range of motion. Flexibility training comprises activities that stretch and lengthen muscles.

These exercises usually start with simpler movements and then progress to more challenging ones as the individual becomes stronger and more flexible. Examples of progressive exercises for strength include bodyweight exercises like squats, lunges, and push-ups. These exercises can be modified by adjusting the number of repetitions or sets, adding resistance with weights or resistance bands, or increasing the range of motion.

For flexibility, progressive exercises may include dynamic stretches like leg swings or arm circles, followed by static stretches held for increasing durations. Individuals can deepen their stretches or incorporate more advanced stretching techniques like proprioceptive neuromuscular facilitation (PNF) stretching as they progress.

The most important aspect of progressive exercises is to start at a suitable level according to the individual's current fitness level and then gradually increase the challenge over time. This helps promote continuous improvement and prevent plateaus.

Some Exercises for Strength and Flexibility

Lunge With a Spinal Twist

It helps to open your hips and increase thoracic (middle back) mobility. It's essential to aid with posture-related pain or for people who sit for an extended period.

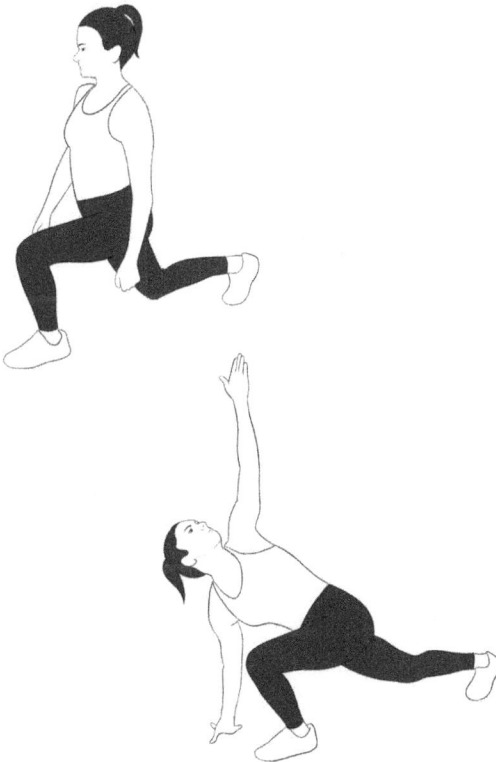

1. Begin by standing with your feet together.

2. Take a wide step forward with your left foot, forming a staggered posture.

3. Bend your left knee and drop into a lunge, keeping your right leg straight behind you and your toes on the ground. You should feel a stretch along the front of your right thighs.

4. Place your right hand on the floor, then twist your upper body to the left while extending your left arm toward the ceiling.

5. Hold for at least 30 seconds.

6. Repeat on the opposite side.

Forward Fold

The primary objective of the forward fold is to stretch the back muscles, hamstrings, and calves while promoting relaxation and release of tension in the spine. This posture also helps improve flexibility in the posterior chain of muscles and increases blood circulation to the brain, enhancing mental clarity.

1. Stand with your feet hip-width apart, knees slightly bent, and arms at your sides.

2. Exhale as you fold forward from the hips, bringing your head to the floor. Tuck your chin under, relax your shoulders, and consider extending the crown of your head to the floor to create a long spine.

3. Keep your knees straight but slightly bent so they are not locked out. This will help protect your back.

4. Use your fingertips to touch the floor. If you feel more comfortable, wrap your arms over your legs.

5. Hold for at least 30 seconds. Remember to breathe.

6. Bend your knees and carefully roll up, beginning with the lower back and stacking one vertebra at a time, to return to standing.

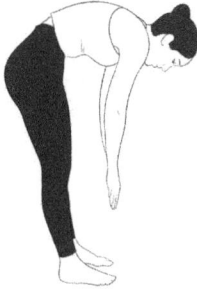

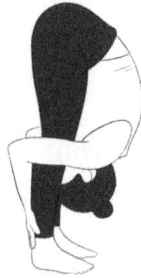

Triceps Stretch

It increases the flexibility of the muscles on the back of your upper arms, plus your neck and shoulders, making it great to do after a chest workout or arms routine.

1. Kneel, sit, or stand tall with feet hip-width apart and arms extended overhead.

2. Bend your right elbow and reach your right hand to touch the top-middle of your back.

3. Reach your left hand overhead and grasp just below your right elbow.

4. Gently pull your right elbow down and toward your head.

5. Hold for at least 30 seconds.

6. Switch arms and repeat.

Tips

- You can start your flexibility training with a gentle stretch and repeat three to five times.

- As your flexibility develops, you will be able to stretch farther with each session.

- Stretching exercises should be done only when your muscles are warm, usually after weightlifting or aerobic sessions.

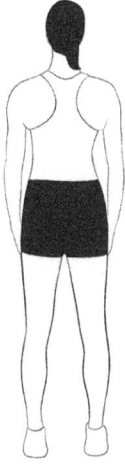

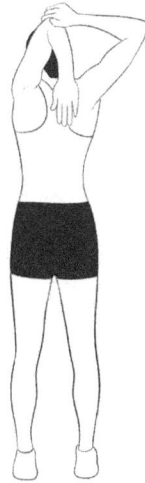

Bodyweight Squat

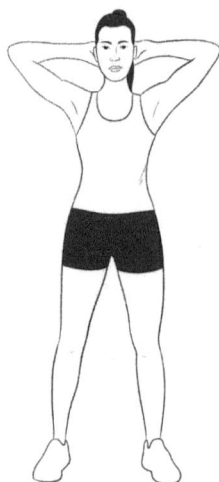

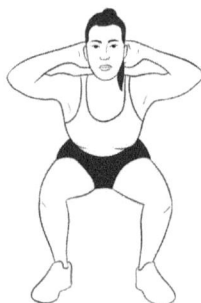

You squat whenever you sit or stand, but don't take this workout for granted. It targets your legs and glutes, the body's most potent muscular group.

Stand with your hands on the back of your head and your feet shoulder-width apart, slightly turned out to open the hip joint.

Lower your body so your thighs are parallel to the floor.

Take a pause and then return to your starting location.

Repeat.

Tips

Avoid placing excessive strain on your knees.

Keep your buttocks pushed out as if preparing to sit on a chair, and engage your hip and thigh muscles to lift yourself.

Ensure that your knees do not protrude forward during the movement; instead, let them move only in the initial phase of the squat, with your hips completing the motion.

A squat can be made more plyometric by hopping from the lowest position back into your starting stance.

Push-Up

Build the muscles in your shoulders and chest with this foundational exercise. To strengthen the muscles in your shoulders and chest:

1. Get down on all fours, placing your hands slightly wider than your shoulders.

2. Straighten your arms and legs.

3. Lower your body until your chest nearly touches the floor.

4. Pause, then push yourself back up.

5. Repeat.

Tips

- If regular push-ups are too complicated, consider doing

them with your knees on the ground. This will lessen the amount of weight you have to lift.

- If basic push-ups are too easy, put your feet on a step or block to enhance the difficulty.

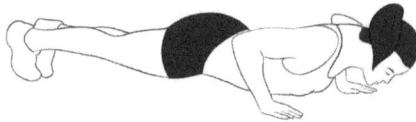

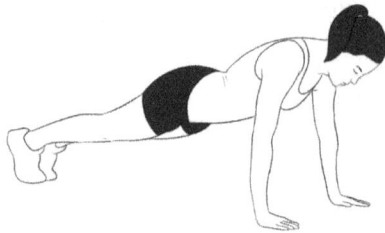

Plank

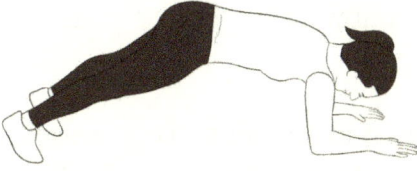

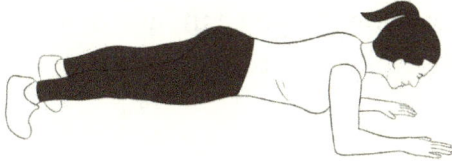

Plank is a common exercise that helps strengthen the core, shoulders, arms, and legs. Plank tones your abdomen and strengthens your upper body. Planks also strengthen the abdominal and lower back muscles at the same time, which might be suitable for persons who suffer from lower back pain.

1. Assume a push-up posture, but bend your arms at the elbows to rest your weight on your forearms.

2. Tighten your core, squeeze your glutes, and maintain a straight body from head to heels.

3. Hold for as long as you can.

Tips

- Plank posture can be painful on your wrists, so we recommend practicing it on your forearm.

- Place your knees on the floor while doing a plank to lessen the weight on your forearms.

Remember to follow the overload principle for progressive exercises!

To gain strength and flexibility, your muscles and joints must be strained and stretched under a higher load than usual. Muscles and joints would be stimulated to adjust to the increased stress. When you stretch a muscle, the muscle fibers or tendons that connect it to the bone grow longer. And as these fibers grow longer, you can improve muscle size during strength and flexibility exercises.

Chapter 7: Integrating Breathwork Into Somatic Practices

Integrating breathwork with somatic practices is mixing conscious breathing techniques with physical motions or exercises to improve awareness, relaxation, and overall well-being. This integration uses the deep connection between the breath and body sensations, emotions, and mental states.

To begin, practitioners usually cultivate mindfulness of the breath, which is generally accomplished through diaphragmatic or deep belly breathing. This fundamental breath awareness assists individuals in developing a consistent and relaxing rhythm, generating a sense of grounding and presence in the moment.

Participants coordinate their breathing with precise movements or exercises as the somatic practice progresses. Breathwork, for example, is synchronized with various positions, or asanas in yoga, to allow for seamless transitions and to strengthen the mind-body connection. Similarly, in qigong or tai chi, practitioners coordinate their breathing with flowing motions to promote energy flow and balance.

The breath guides the somatic exercise, providing important feedback on one's bodily and emotional states. Individuals who pay attention to the quality and depth of their breath can find areas of tension or resistance in their bodies and thus experiment with techniques to release or soften them.

Furthermore, incorporating breathing exercises into somatic activities improves the efficacy of relaxation therapies. Practitioners can stimulate the body's relaxation response by actively regulating their breath, resulting in decreased tension, a lower heart rate, and improved mental clarity. Techniques like progressive muscle relaxation or body scanning can be combined with rhythmic breathing patterns to deepen and encourage relaxation.

Incorporating breathwork with somatic activities provides a comprehensive approach to health and wellness by exploiting the close relationship between breath, body, and mind. By practicing conscious breathing, individuals can improve their somatic experiences, increase self-awareness, and create inner balance and harmony.

Breathing Exercises for Relaxation

Here are some breathing exercises for relaxation:

Box Breathing

It is an easy approach to slowing down in the moment. Each breathing phrase is completed for an equal number of counts, similar to the sides of a square. It is used to reduce stress, enhance relaxation, and support mental health.

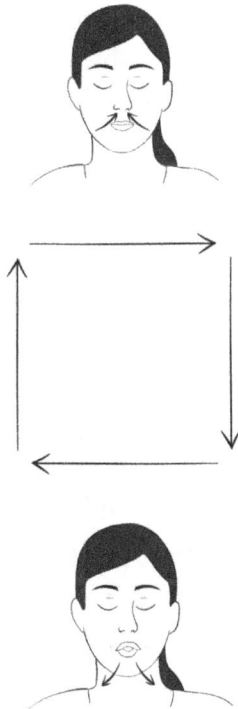

1. Inhale for four counts.

2. Hold your breath in for four counts.

3. Exhale for four counts.

4. After the exhale, hold your breath for four counts before starting again.

5. Repeat for 3 to 6 cycles.

Equal Breathing

Sama Vritti, or equal breathing, is a breathing technique focused on keeping your inhales and exhales equal in length. It helps to choose an appropriate breath length that is neither too simple nor too challenging while also being quick enough to remain consistent throughout the practice. This typically lies between three and five counts. This technique is used to reduce the high blood pressure of seniors and may enhance mental health and increase oxygen delivery to the brain and lungs.

1. Choose a comfortable sitting position.

2. Breathe in and out of your nose.

3. Count each breath and exhale to ensure they are equal in duration. Alternatively, select a word or brief phrase to repeat with each inhalation and exhalation.

4. If you feel comfortable, add a little pause for breath retention after each inhalation and exhalation (normal breathing includes a natural pause).

5. Continue to practice this breathing for at least five minutes.

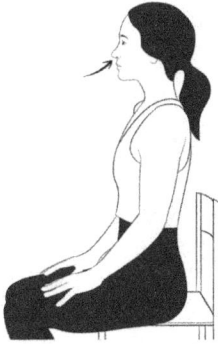

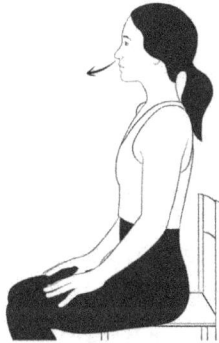

Deep Breathing

Deep breathing relieves shortness of breath by preventing air from becoming stuck in your lungs, allowing you to breathe in fresh air. It may help you feel more relaxed and focused and is used to lower blood pressure and heart rate, reduce levels of stress hormones in the blood, reduce lactic acid build-up in muscle tissue, balance levels of oxygen and carbon dioxide in the blood, improve immune system functioning, increase physical energy, and increase feelings of calm and well-being.

1. While standing or sitting, pull your elbows back slightly

to allow your chest to expand.

2. Take a deep breath via the nose.

3. Hold your breath for a count of five.

4. Slowly exhale through your nose.

Tips

- Choose a place to do your breathing exercise. It could be in your bed, on your living room floor, or in a comfortable chair.
- Don't force it. This can make you feel more stressed.
- Try to do it at the same time once or twice a day.
- Wear comfortable clothes.
- Many breathing exercises take only a few minutes. If you have more time, you can do them for 10 minutes or more to get even greater benefits

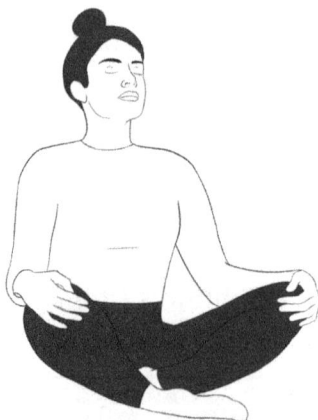

Syncing Breath With Movements

Breathing in sync with movement involves coordinating inhalation and exhalation with specific physical actions or transitions. This practice can help to improve mindfulness and energy flow and promote a sense of ease in the body. You can stay more present and mindful during physical activity by connecting breath and movement.

Being aware of your natural breath rhythm is essential to incorporate breath synchronization. Start by observing how your breath moves in and out without trying to control it. This helps you establish a baseline for your breath pattern and is a reference point for syncing your breath with movements.

After becoming aware of your breath pattern, you can start coordinating your inhalations and exhalations with specific movements. In yoga, for example, inhalations may coincide with movements that expand the body, while exhalations may align with movements that contract or fold the body.

It is essential to synchronize breath and movement seamlessly, ensuring a smooth transition between the two. Try to maintain a steady and rhythmic breath pattern and avoid forced or strained breathing. This synchronicity can enhance the mind-body connection, allowing you to move with greater awareness and precision while conserving energy and reducing tension.

Syncing breath with movements can also promote relaxation and reduce stress by activating the body's relaxation response. Deep, diaphragmatic breathing during movement can help regulate the autonomic nervous system, leading to decreased heart rate, blood pressure, and muscle tension. This can result in a more enjoyable and fulfilling practice.

Syncing breath with movements is a powerful tool for enhancing mindfulness and promoting holistic well-being. Connecting your breath and movement can cultivate a more profound sense of presence, vitality, and connection within your body.

How to Sync Breath With Movement

When we inhale, we breathe down and out, which stabilizes the spine by increasing pressure. This inhalation phase is the eccentric, or lengthening, portion of our breathing pattern, allowing us to stretch and build tension in the abdominal cavity. It generates energy and pressure for the abdominal cavity to recoil. On the other hand, exhalations involve breathing up and in, activating muscles to stabilize the spine further. This phase is the concentric, or shortening, portion of our breathing pattern, where we either release the gathered energy or use it for exertion. In summary, inhalations increase tension and energy, while exhalations release tension or use it for movement recoil.

During Inhalation

During the eccentric phase of movement, we should synchronize with inhalation or the eccentric phase of breathing. This applies when moving with gravity or resistance, such as lowering in a squat, deadlift, or pull-up. Optionally, inhaling at the top of the movement can increase pressure in the abdominal cavity to stabilize the spine, or inhaling throughout the descent is also viable. Each option has its pros and cons.

Inhale at the Top and Hold Your Breath on the Way Down

- Generates the most pressure to stabilize the spine, suitable for heavy lifts and external loads
- Particularly effective for maximizing strength during lifts
- Not advisable for individuals with a compromised pelvic floor or abdominal wall, such as during pregnancy and early postpartum due to high pressure

Inhale Throughout the Entire Descent

- Generates less pressure to stabilize the spine
- Helps manage pressure within the abdominal cavity in a controlled manner
- More suitable for exercises with decreased loading rather than maximum lifts
- Offers a safer approach for individuals with pelvic floor or abdominal wall issues

During Exhalation

During the concentric phase of movement, exhaling is crucial, especially when moving against gravity or resistance. This includes jumping from a squat, lifting a bar in a deadlift, or pulling up towards a bar. Exhaling during this phase helps to exert force and facilitate movement. There are variations in exhalation timing, and it can occur at the bottom to aid in recoiling out of the squat, throughout the entire movement, or at the end of the movement.

Exhaling at the Bottom or Throughout the Movement

- Exhaling at the bottom or throughout the movement releases energy accumulated from inhalations, aiding in recoiling from the bottom of the movement.

- Exhaling up and in with the pelvic floor and abs helps manage pressure in the abdominal cavity, which is crucial during pregnancy and early postpartum to prevent issues like prolapse or worsened diastasis recti.

Holding the Breath Throughout the Movement

- Holding the breath maintains intra-abdominal pressure from inhalations, stabilizing the spine during heavy lifts and external loads.

- Pressure loss during heavy lifts can compromise form and increase the risk of injury (Conley, 2019).

Mindful Breathing for Stress Reduction

Mindful breathing is a technique that reduces stress and promotes relaxation by focusing on the breath and bringing awareness to the present moment. In today's fast-paced society, chronic stress can take a toll on both physical and emotional health, leading to conditions like burnout, depression, and anxiety.

Mindful breathing exercises offer a simple yet effective way to manage stress levels and promote well-being. By taking just 5–10 minutes a day to find a quiet space, relax, and focus on breathing, individuals can bring their bodies to a state of balance and reduce the harmful effects of stress.

To practice mindful breathing, find a quiet and comfortable place to sit or lie down. Close your eyes and take a few deep breaths to settle into the present moment. Then, bring your attention to your breath, noticing either the sensation of the air entering and leaving your nostrils or the rise and fall of your chest and abdomen. As you breathe in, mentally note "inhaling," and as you breathe out, note "exhaling."

If your mind wanders, gently bring your focus back to your breath without judgment. With regular practice, mindful breathing can improve focus, regulate emotions, and increase self-awareness, providing a valuable tool for maintaining overall health and resilience. Some mindful breathing techniques are listed below (Rae Ackerman, 2023).

Breath Awareness Meditation

Breath awareness meditation is a mindful breathing exercise that can help you enhance your attention, reduce tension and anxiety, and achieve overall calmness. The primary goal is to prevent passing thoughts and emotions while focusing entirely on breathing.

1. Find an alert, comfortable position on a chair, floor cushion, or bench.

2. Sit with your spine erect.

3. Bring your attention to the natural sensations of the breath in the body.

4. Don't try to control your breath. It doesn't matter if it is short and shallow or long and deep.

5. Try to follow the breath through complete cycles, from the beginning of an inhalation to the end of an exhalation and then on to the next cycle.

6. Thoughts may enter the mind. This is natural. Simply allow them to arise and pass.

7. If a chain of thought hijacks your attention and you lose awareness of the breath, gently return your attention to the sensations of breathing.

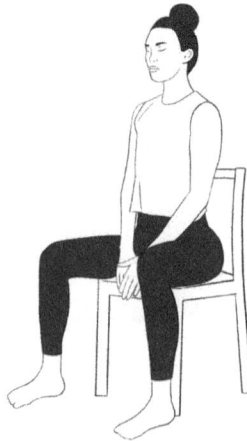

Pursed-Lip Breathing

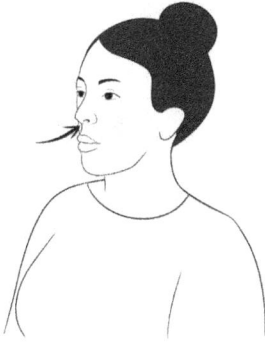

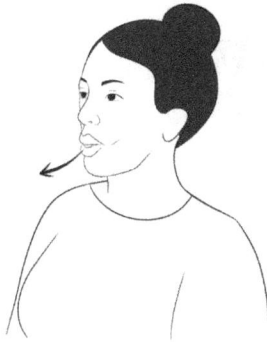

Pursed-lip breathing is a simple controlled breathing technique that can help ease anxiety symptoms. This approach is a wonderful way to relax and can also assist those with respiratory issues improve lung function.

1. Begin by inhaling slowly through your nose for approximately two seconds.

2. Next, purse or pucker your lips like you're blowing out a candle.

3. Finally, exhale slowly through pursed lips for around four seconds.

Mindful Slow and Deep Breathing

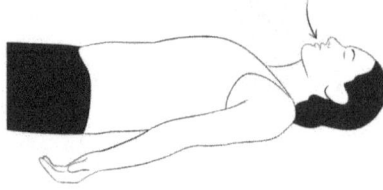

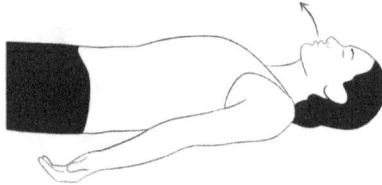

You can start introducing mindful change once you're comfortable with mindful breathing. The following methods guide you toward a soothing, stress-reducing breath that prevents over-breathing.

1. Ideally, do this exercise lying down to allow the diaphragm to move more freely.

2. Start by taking a few typical, regular-sized breaths.

3. When ready, inhale deeply, then exhale fully and gently until the lungs are completely empty. Breathing out with pursed lips can help you reach the optimal ratio of 60% expiration to 40% inhalation.

4. Instead of breathing via your chest, breathe in and out through your abdomen. Consider it like a balloon filling and flowing out.

5. Repeat steps 3 and 4 for five minutes, focusing on the sensation of breathing in and out of the body.

6. If you find it difficult to relax, let go of relaxation as an objective and concentrate solely on breathing.

7. Begin by practicing this technique for five minutes daily, gradually increasing to 10 minutes over the following weeks.

Tips

- Schedule a specific time during the day to practice these methods, and set reminders on your phone or other devices to help you remember.

- Start by gradually experimenting with different breathing techniques until you find the one that works best.

- Once you've identified the most effective method for managing your anxiety, aim to incorporate it into your daily routine to prevent nervousness.

- Keep a log of your symptoms before and during each breathing exercise, and stop if you experience any unpleasant symptoms. If you have concerns, consider consulting a healthcare professional.

Chapter 8: Building a Community Through Somatic Practices

Building a community through somatic practices involves establishing a welcoming environment where individuals may explore and participate in various somatic exercises and activities. This community-centered practice promotes connections, well-being, and personal development.

Inclusivity is vital to somatic community building, ensuring that people of diverse backgrounds, skills, and experiences feel accepted and appreciated. This includes providing a wide range of seminars and workshops that suit various interests and needs and maintaining a secure and courteous environment where everyone feels heard and valued.

Collaboration is vital since it encourages people to share their expertise, experiences, and thoughts. This can include group talks, peer assistance, and activities where individuals work together towards common goals. By cultivating a sense of belonging and collaboration, community members can learn from each other and support one another's growth and development.

Building a community entails cultivating a sense of shared purpose and connection. This can be accomplished through common rituals, customs, and activities that foster group unity and cohesion. For example, community members may meet regularly for group meditation sessions, mindfulness practices, or movement exercises, fostering a sense of shared intention and energy.

Furthermore, fostering community through somatic practices demands continual communication and participation with participants. This could include regular check-ins, feedback sessions, and chances for community members to share their ideas and proposals for future activities and events. By actively incorporating participants in decision-making, community leaders can ensure that the community remains responsive to its members' needs and interests.

Overall, somatic practices help create a friendly and inclusive environment where people can connect, grow, and thrive together. Somatic communities can help people explore their bodies, minds, and spirits in meaningful and transformative ways by cultivating a sense of belonging, collaboration, and shared purpose (Deasy, 2014; Rasmussen et al., 2021).

Group Participation Exercises

Group participation exercises in somatic therapy encourage individuals to connect and promote healing within a group setting. These exercises focus on facilitating communication, building trust, and fostering a sense of community among participants. Here are some examples of group participation exercises commonly used in somatic therapy.

Body Scan Meditation

Participants are guided through a relaxation exercise where they systematically focus on different body parts, noticing sensations and letting go of tension. This exercise promotes mindfulness and helps individuals become more attuned to their bodily experiences.

Partner Stretching

Participants work in pairs to gently stretch and support each other's bodies. This exercise encourages trust and cooperation while promoting physical relaxation and flexibility.

Mirror Exercises

Participants pair up and take turns mirroring each other's movements and gestures. This exercise fosters empathy, nonverbal communication, and attunement to others' body language.

Group Breathing Exercises

Participants engage in synchronized breathing exercises, such as deep belly breathing or box breathing. This activity promotes relaxation, coherence, and a sense of unity among group members.

Guided Movement Exploration

Participants are led through guided movements and explorations, allowing them to experiment with different ways of moving and expressing themselves. This exercise encourages creativity, self-expression, and body awareness.

Circle Sharing

Participants gather in a circle and take turns sharing their thoughts, feelings, and experiences related to a specific topic or theme. This exercise promotes vulnerability, empathy, and social support within the group.

Grounding and Centering Practices

Participants engage in grounding and centering exercises, such as mindful walking or body-based visualizations. These practices help individuals feel more present, connected, and anchored in their bodies and the present moment.

Overall, group participation exercises in somatic therapy provide opportunities for individuals to connect, explore, and heal together in a supportive and collaborative environment. These exercises promote embodied awareness, interpersonal connection, and holistic well-being within the group context (Robinson, 2020; Ph.D., 2023).

Some Group Exercises

Following are some exercises that you can perform in pairs.

Partner Forward Fold

The Forward Fold pose stretches the hamstrings, calves, and back. Doing a Forward Fold in your partner's yoga practice can provide an even deeper stretch and can be done seated or standing.

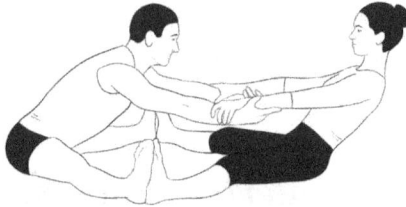

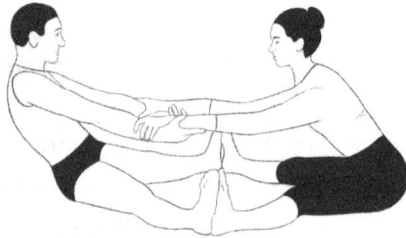

1. To perform a seated Partner Forward Fold, face your partner and straddle your legs.

2. Then, lean forward and clasp your partner's hands, rocking back and forth so that each person feels the stretch.

3. To make the pose easier, bend your knees slightly or broaden your stance. Start from a seated pike rather than a straddle position to make it more intense.

4. You and your partner will be about one foot apart if you are standing.

5. Bend forward slowly from the hips, relaxing your back and extending your chest as far as possible to the floor.

6. Grab your partner's arms and bring them closer together to deepen the stretch.

7. Keep your knees slightly bent and your hands on your quads to reduce the impact of the stretch.

Four-Person Plank

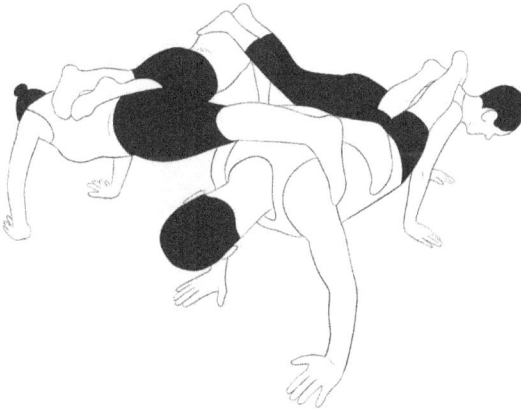

1. Gather four people of similar heights and fitness levels on a flat surface.

2. The first pair will enter the plank position by lying face down on the ground and holding themselves up with their forearms and toes. Their elbows should be squarely beneath their shoulders, and their bodies should be in a straight line from head to feet. This is the start position for the workout.

3. The remaining pair will stand behind the first pair, close together. Each participant in the second pair will place their forearms on the backs of the people in the first pair. Their elbows should be bent about 90 degrees, and their hands clasped together.

4. Focus on appropriate alignment and stability, working the leg, core, and gluteal muscles.

5. Hold for a predetermined time, beginning at at least 30 seconds.

6. Use verbal signals to promote teamwork and motivation.

7. Then, gently drop down, rest, and extend your core, chest, shoulders, and hips.

Temple Pose

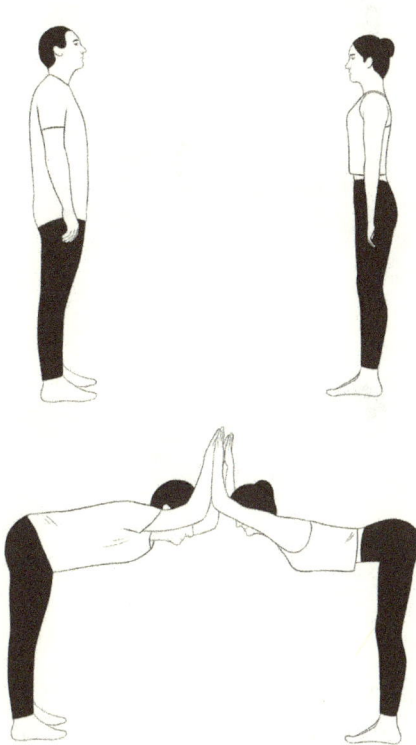

Temple Pose is a simple two-person yoga pose that deep stretches both partners' chests and shoulders.

1. Begin facing each other a few feet away, with your feet hip-width apart.

2. Inhale, raise your hands overhead and begin to bend at the hips.

3. Lean forward until you meet your partner's hands, then continue until your forearms and elbows are in contact.

4. Press into your partner to deepen the stretch through your chest, keeping a tiny arch in your back.

Partner Boat Pose

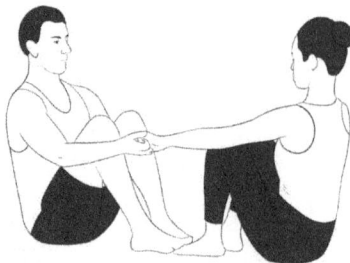

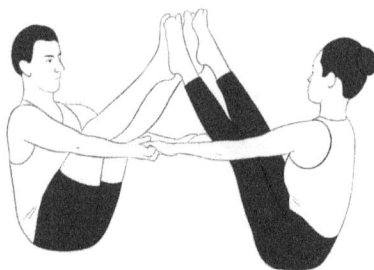

Boat pose is a balancing posture that partners may find easy to perform. If done correctly, your bodies will form a W in the air.

1. You will begin seated with your knees bent, facing your partner, feet flat on the floor, and toes touching.

2. Grab hands and lift one leg at a time into the air, pressing into your partner's foot.

3. When the soles of your feet touch your partner's, slowly straighten one leg at a time until both legs are erect in the air.

4. Your hamstrings and shoulders should feel stretched out.

5. For an added challenge, attempt this pose with your legs wide open.

Fostering Connection and Shared Well-Being

Fostering connection and shared well-being is essential in any group setting, including somatic therapy sessions. Facilitators can incorporate various practices and activities to build trust, empathy, and a sense of community among participants. Here are some strategies for fostering connection and shared well-being using somatic therapy:

- Start each session with icebreaker activities that allow participants to introduce themselves, share a little about their background, and connect personally. This helps create a welcoming atmosphere and encourages openness and unity.

- Incorporate partner exercises that involve physical contact, such as partner stretching or massage techniques. These activities promote trust, cooperation, and mutual support among participants, fostering a sense of connection and shared experience.

- Create opportunities for group-sharing circles where participants can express themselves, share their thoughts and feelings, and listen to others in a supportive and nonjudgmental environment. Encourage active listening, empathy, and validation of each other's experiences.

- Integrate mindful communication practices into the sessions, such as active listening, compassionate speaking, and nonverbal cues. Encourage participants to communicate with authenticity, empathy, and respect for each other's perspectives.

- Movement explorations are where participants engage in group movement activities, improvisations, or dance exercises. This allows individuals to connect with each other through shared movement experiences, promoting a sense of unity and interconnectedness.

- Provide time for reflection and integration at the end of each session, allowing participants to process their experiences, insights, and emotions. Encourage group members to share their reflections and support each other in integrating somatic practices into their daily lives.

- Create a safe and inclusive environment where all participants feel valued, respected, and heard. Set clear ground rules for communication and behavior, and address any issues or conflicts that arise with sensitivity and compassion.

By incorporating these strategies into somatic therapy sessions, facilitators can nurture a sense of connection, belonging, and shared well-being among participants, fostering a supportive and transformative group experience (Lucini & Pagani, 2021; Granero-Jiménez et al., 2022).

Feedback Mechanism for Continuous Improvement

When providing feedback in somatic therapy, it's important to create a system that will help improve the effectiveness of the interventions, increase client satisfaction, and promote continuing growth. Below are the steps to implement such a system:

1. Give clients organized forms to fill out with questions about their satisfaction with the session, the success of the

treatment used, and the connection between the therapist and the client.

2. Schedule regular check-in sessions with clients to discuss their progress, obstacles, and overall satisfaction with the therapy process. This can happen during or after sessions.

3. Periodically conduct anonymous surveys to gather feedback from clients who prefer to share their opinions anonymously. The survey should cover aspects of the therapy process, including the therapist's approach, the perceived benefits of the sessions, and areas for improvement.

4. Therapists should reflect and identify areas for growth by reviewing session recordings, seeking feedback from colleagues or supervisors, and attending professional development workshops.

5. Hold peer supervision sessions where therapists can discuss their cases, share insights, and receive constructive feedback from their colleagues.

6. Use standardized outcome measures to evaluate the efficacy of somatic therapy and monitor client progress over time. These measures may include validated evaluation instruments for symptoms, functional disability, and quality of life.

7. Create quality improvement initiatives within somatic therapy practices or organizations to assess and enhance treatment performance. This may involve conducting root cause analysis of any issues or complaints, executing corrective activities, and monitoring results.

8. Prioritize a client-centered approach to therapy where the client's feedback and preferences are recognized and included in the therapeutic process. This promotes successful therapy outcomes by increasing client participation.

A comprehensive feedback mechanism for continuous improvement enhances satisfaction and achieves better therapeutic outcomes over time (Dallaway et al., 2022; Trewick et al., 2022).

Chapter 9: Case Studies and Success Stories

There are a lot of people out there who are benefiting from somatic therapy. People have shared how it has helped them deal with various physical and emotional issues, by focusing on the mind-body connection and addressing underlying patterns of tension, stress, and trauma stored in the body.

Somatic therapy offers a holistic approach to healing and well-being. Through gentle hands-on techniques, guided movement exercises, breathwork, and mindfulness practices, somatic therapy helps individuals release muscular tension, improve mobility, reduce pain, and enhance overall body awareness.

Here are some real-life stories of people who experienced profound effects on their mental and emotional health through somatic therapy which helped them process and integrate past experiences, regulate their emotions, and cultivate a greater sense of resilience and self-compassion. Here are some case studies and success stories of people benefiting from somatic therapy

I. Case Study: John's Journey Towards Healing Through Somatic Therapy

Patient's Background

John is an 80-year-old man who has been struggling with mobility issues and chronic pain in his hips and knees for the past few years. His mobility has gradually declined due to osteoarthritis and stiffness in his joints, making it difficult for him to perform daily activities such as walking, climbing stairs, and getting in and out of chairs. John has also experienced feelings of frustration, isolation, and depression as a result of his physical limitations.

Somatic Therapy Approach

John decides to explore somatic therapy as a complementary approach to managing his mobility issues and chronic pain. He meets with a certified somatic therapist who works with seniors to improve movement, reduce pain, and enhance overall well-being. During the initial assessment, the therapist evaluates John's posture, gait, range of motion, and muscular tension or restriction areas.

Based on the assessment findings, the therapist develops a tailored somatic therapy plan for John, focusing on restoring mobility, increasing body awareness, and reducing pain. The plan includes gentle hands-on techniques, guided movement exercises, breathwork, and relaxation techniques.

Treatment Progress

Throughout several sessions, John begins to experience noticeable improvements in his mobility and pain levels. The therapist helps John release muscle tension and improve joint mobility through hands-on manipulation and guided movement explorations. John learns to move more quickly and efficiently, allowing him to perform daily activities with less effort and discomfort.

Additionally, the therapist teaches John various self-care strategies to help him manage his pain and maintain his mobility between sessions. John learns to perform simple movement exercises, stretches, and breathing techniques at home to alleviate tension and improve his overall well-being. With consistent practice, John becomes more confident in his ability to move and engage in activities that were once challenging for him.

Outcome

After completing a series of Somatic Therapy sessions, John experiences significant improvements in his mobility, pain levels, and overall quality of life. He is able to walk longer distances, climb stairs more efficiently, and participate in activities that he enjoys with greater comfort and freedom. John also reports feeling less isolated and depressed, as he can engage more fully in social interactions and recreational pursuits.

By incorporating somatic therapy into his routine, John has gained greater control over his health and well-being as a senior. Somatic therapy has provided him with a holistic approach to managing his mobility issues and chronic pain, allowing him to maintain his independence and enjoy a more active and fulfilling lifestyle in his later years (Rothberg, 2014).

II. Case Study: Lilly's Journey to Healing Through Somatic Therapy

Patient Background

Lilly, a 50-year-old retired teacher, has been struggling with chronic anxiety and depression for several years. Despite trying various medications and traditional talk therapy, she finds little relief from her symptoms and often feels disconnected from her body. Lilly's anxiety manifests as tightness in her chest, shallow breathing, and a constant sense of agitation, while her depression leaves her feeling emotionally numb and fatigued.

Somatic Therapy Approach

Seeking a different approach to healing, Lilly decides to explore Somatic Therapy. Working with a somatic therapist, Lilly begins to explore the connection between her physical sensations and her emotional state. Through gentle movement exercises, breath work, and hands-on techniques, Lilly learns to identify and release the tension stored in her body, allowing her to experience a greater sense of relaxation and ease.

As Lilly continues her somatic therapy sessions, she notices profound shifts in her mental and emotional well-being. She becomes more attuned to her body's signals and learns to respond to them with compassion and curiosity rather than judgment. Over time, Lilly's anxiety and depression begin to lift, and she feels more present, grounded, and alive.

Outcome

One of the most transformative aspects of Lilly's somatic therapy journey was learning to trust her body's innate wisdom. Through somatic therapy, Lilly discovered that her body held valuable insights and resources for healing that she had previously overlooked. By reconnecting with her body and honoring its messages, Lilly cultivated a deep sense of self-awareness and resilience that supported her on her path to recovery.

Today, Lilly continues to practice Somatic Therapy as part of her self-care routine, using the techniques she learned to navigate life's challenges with greater ease and grace. Somatic therapy has not only helped Lilly alleviate her symptoms of anxiety and depression but has also empowered her to live a more vibrant, fulfilling life in her golden years (Rothberg, 2014).

Real Life Stories

Eve's Success Story

Eva shared her story, how somatic therapy completely transformed her life. A few years back, she was drowning in stress and anxiety. she was working crazy hours as a manager in a tech company, dealing with difficult employees and struggling to meet the sky-high expectations. Panic attacks became a regular occurrence, leaving her terrified and sleepless at night, always worried for the next day.

But then she found somatic therapy, and it was like a beacon of hope in her darkest moments. her therapist helped her delve into the root causes of her anxiety, tracing it back to childhood feelings of inadequacy and the need to please others constantly. Through somatic therapy and mindfulness techniques, she successfully learned to confront and release these deep-seated fears. She stated:

> As I progressed in therapy, I began to notice a shift in my mindset. The grip of anxiety loosened, and my perfectionist tendencies started to fade away. I realized that I didn't have to sacrifice my health and happiness for success in my career. With the support of my therapist, I decided to work less and prioritize self-care.

> And let me tell you, the transformation was remarkable. I reconnected with old friends, embraced new hobbies like yoga and writing, and finally started enjoying life again. My sleep improved, the panic attacks became less frequent, and I felt more grounded and centered.

Somatic therapy gave me the tools to navigate through life's challenges with grace and resilience. It taught me to listen to my body, honor my emotions, and cultivate inner peace. Today, I'm living proof that healing is possible, even amid chaos. (Stora, 2023)

Mary's Journey to Emotional Healing

Mary, a 66-year-old widow, had been grappling with grief and loneliness following the loss of her husband. She found it challenging to cope with her emotions and often felt overwhelmed by sadness and despair. Seeking support, Mary began attending somatic therapy sessions, where she learned to connect with her body's sensations and express her emotions through movement. Through somatic exercises and compassionate guidance from her therapist, Mary gradually processed her grief and found a sense of peace and acceptance. She credits somatic therapy with helping her navigate her emotional journey and rediscover joy in life (Somatic Experiencing International).

Thorgal's Success Story

I've had ten sessions so far over the past six months. Before that, I was doing Traditional psychotherapy for the past three years. While I felt the progress with psychotherapy was very slow after two years and still felt my mind stuck and traumatized with recurrent high anxiety fits, Somatic Experiencing has been a game changer.

I feel like my mind is learning to get back to normal, to snap out of this permanent rigid and tense state, bracing for the next painful blow life will deal to me, and that I will overreact and suffer more than necessary because of it. As a result, I'm getting better socially and smoother at work, too; I can better express myself and temper my emotional reactions. It feels like my inner wounded child is finally getting the nurturing, non-judgmental, and patient attention, the mental space it has lacked all its life to heal and grow up eventually. I'm 37, by the way.

Meanwhile, it has not been an easy process. I've had to go through very dark and uncomfortable sessions, and sometimes we couldn't complete them, even taking 2 hours, so I would walk out feeling very sad or cold. But other times, we could complete the emotional processing of some traumas, and I've walked out feeling so light and liberated.

I would like to add that you don't have to have been in war, a car incident, or a victim of violent or sexual aggression to be traumatized. I suffer more from complex traumas, C-PTSD. The result of long-lasting destructive conditions and social dynamics in my family was barely noticeable to an outsider. This had left me damaged on a level that nobody around me could understand except therapists who just saw I was obviously hurt. Everybody around me to whom I would open up about my social issues would tell me to "just change my thoughts" to read this article or watch this video about personal or spiritual development.

While it might have worked for them because they were either less damaged or damaged in a different way than me, it didn't bring me many benefits to follow their advice. Over time, every time I would hear the same useless advice from people willing to help on a very superficial level but unequipped, it became increasingly frustrating and painful. Basically, I felt gaslighted; if this advice didn't work with me, then it was just my fault. I didn't try hard enough, meditate enough, don't do breathing exercises enough, etc... Somatic Experiencing has been liberating me from this. (Thorgal256, 2020)

Robert's Anxiety Relief

I am a 60-year-old retiree who has suffered from acute anxiety for most of my life. My anxiousness appeared as racing thoughts, trouble sleeping, and regular panic attacks. Despite trying several drugs and talk therapy, I experienced no alleviation from my symptoms. Desperate for a solution, I decided to try somatic therapy. I learned to control my nervous system and calm my anxious thoughts through breathwork, mindfulness, and body awareness exercises. I gradually reduced my anxiety levels and learned how to manage my symptoms successfully (Rothberg, 2014).

These examples show how somatic therapy can help seniors by addressing various physical, emotional, and psychological difficulties, enhancing their overall health and quality of life.

Testimonials

From Sarah:

Somatic therapy has been a game-changer for me. I struggled with chronic pain and emotional trauma for years, and traditional talk therapy just didn't seem to cut it. But through somatic therapy, I learned to reconnect with my body and release the tension and stored emotions trapped within. It's been a journey of healing and self-discovery, and I'm forever grateful for the profound impact it's had on my life. (Fluent Body, 2024)

From James:

I was skeptical at first, but somatic therapy completely exceeded my expectations. I had been battling anxiety and depression for years, and I felt stuck in a cycle of negative thought patterns. Somatic therapy helped me break free from that cycle by teaching me to listen to my body's signals and process my emotions in a healthy way. It's been incredibly empowering to reclaim control over my mental and emotional well-being. (Somatic Healing Therapy, 2024)

From Maya:

As a survivor of trauma, I was hesitant to try therapy again after previous experiences left me feeling unheard and invalidated. However, somatic therapy offered me a safe and nurturing space to explore my trauma and heal at my own pace. Through gentle movement, breathwork, and mindfulness practices, I've been able to release the pent-up tension and fear stored in my body. Somatic therapy has truly been a lifeline on my journey toward healing and wholeness. (Somatic Experiencing Therapy)

From Alex:

Somatic therapy has been a revelation for me. I've struggled with body image issues and disordered eating for as long as I can remember, but somatic therapy helped me cultivate a deeper sense of self-compassion and acceptance. By tuning into the sensations and emotions present in my body, I've been able to break free from harmful patterns and nourish a more loving relationship with myself. It's been a transformative experience that has touched every aspect of my life. (Somatic Therapy Partners, 2024)

From Patrick:

After grappling with daily flashbacks stemming from a violent attack for two decades, I turned to Somatic Experiencing therapy. Through multiple sessions, my body gradually processed the long-held trauma, and my mind regained trust in my physical self. Since completing the initial sessions, I haven't encountered flashbacks in the same debilitating manner as before; instead, the traumatic event feels like a distant memory. Unlike traditional talk therapy, which I had previously tried, Somatic Experiencing therapy provided a safe space for me to address the stored trauma in my body rather than solely focusing on verbal recounting. I highly recommend SE therapy to individuals dealing with flashbacks, nightmares, or physical symptoms related to past trauma. It has been transformative for me, and I continue to apply the techniques learned in therapy for self-care and mental well-being. (Somatic Experiencing International, 2024)

From Angelena:

The method of Somatic Experiencing to help me relieve stored trauma works. SE gets to the root cause of my emotional challenges. I did talk therapy, and though it did serve a purpose at the time, nothing compares to the emotional release of the Somatic Experiencing method. I recommend this method for anyone on the healing of emotional trauma. (Somatic Healing Therapy, 2024)

Outcomes

Somatic therapy can provide various outcomes depending on the individual's specific needs and aspirations. Some possible effects of somatic therapy are

- Reduced trauma symptoms: Somatic treatment can help people process and release stored trauma in their bodies, resulting in fewer symptoms like flashbacks, nightmares, hypervigilance, and emotional dysregulation.
- Improved emotional regulation: Learning to connect with physical sensations and regulate the nervous system can help people improve their emotional regulation and feel more peaceful and stable.

- Increased body awareness: Somatic therapy encourages people to become more aware of their bodily feelings, which helps them better comprehend and respond to their physical and emotional needs.

- Improved stress management: Learning somatic skills for relaxing, grounding, and self-soothing can help people manage stress more efficiently and develop resilience in life's obstacles.

- Improved interpersonal relationships: As people become more aware of their bodies and emotions, they may create a better understanding and compassion for others, resulting in more pleasant and rewarding interactions.

- Increased self-confidence and empowerment: Somatic therapy can help people take control of their healing process and make suitable changes in their lives, giving them a sense of agency.

- Overall well-being and quality of life: Somatic therapy, which addresses both physical and emotional health components, can help enhance overall well-being and quality of life.

These results are frequently obtained through experiential exercises, mindfulness practices, body-oriented techniques, and supportive therapy interactions tailored to each individual's specific needs and goals (Araminta, 2021; Krouse, 2023).

Conclusion

This thorough guide to somatic therapy for seniors has shed light on the importance of dealing with stress, trauma, and healing in later life. Individuals can better appreciate the potential benefits of somatic therapy for improving well-being and quality of life if they understand the principles behind it and how they apply to seniors.

The consequences of stress on seniors, both physical and mental, have been carefully investigated, emphasizing the importance of stress reduction strategies such as breathwork, relaxation, and mindful movement sequences. Furthermore, the acknowledgment of trauma symptoms and the function of somatic therapy in trauma recovery emphasize the significance of holistic approaches to dealing with past traumas in later life.

We hope the practical somatic exercises in this guide will provide seniors with a wide range of options for improving strength, flexibility, and general vitality. Integrating breathwork with somatic activities improves stress reduction and mindfulness, giving elders important tools for self-care and resilience. Somatic practices encourage connection and shared well-being, resulting in supportive situations where elders can thrive and grow.

We've seen real-world examples of seniors benefiting from somatic therapy through case studies and success stories, demonstrating these techniques' transformative potential in increasing quality of life and fostering holistic healing. Testimonies and outcomes speak to the success of somatic therapy in resolving a wide range of physical and mental issues experienced by seniors, highlighting its importance as a comprehensive approach to well-being in later life.

Finally, this guide is a comprehensive resource for seniors who want to learn more about the transforming power of somatic therapy in promoting health, healing, and well-being in later life. Seniors who embrace and integrate somatic practices into their everyday lives can create resilience, vitality, and a greater connection with themselves and others, improving their overall quality of life.

Recap of Key Concepts

I. An Overview of Somatic Therapy for Seniors

- Somatic therapy emphasizes the mind-body connection and uses experiential activities to reduce stress and trauma and promote healing.
- It is essential for seniors since it addresses age-related concerns and promotes overall well-being in later years.

II. Understanding Somatic Therapy

- Somatic therapy focuses on bodily awareness, mindfulness, and movement to promote healing and reduce stress.
- Its importance to seniors stems from its ability to manage physical and mental concerns typical in later life.

III. Effects of Stress on Seniors

- Stress can worsen age-related health issues and lower quality of life.
- Identifying frequent stressors in aging and implementing stress-reduction measures are critical for fostering well-being.

IV. Trauma in Later Life

- Seniors may endure a range of traumas, including historical, loss, and medical trauma.
- Recognizing trauma symptoms and understanding the role of somatic therapy in trauma healing is critical for dealing with past experiences and facilitating healing.

V. Somatic Approaches to Stress Reduction

- Somatic therapy focuses on mind-body connection and breathwork techniques to reduce stress.
- Integrating breathwork with movement and mindful movement sequences might help seniors relax and feel better overall.

VI. Somatic Exercises for Elders

- Various exercises designed for elders increase strength, flexibility, and physical health.
- Interactive components like QR codes and internet materials improve the accessibility and involvement with somatic activities.

VII. Integrating Breathwork With Somatic Practices

- Relaxation breathing techniques and breath-to-movement synchronization assist elders in managing stress and improving mindfulness.

- Mindful breathing exercises are helpful tools for seniors to reduce stress and improve general well-being.

VIII. Building a Community Through Somatic Practices

- Group engagement and connection encourage shared well-being and ongoing improvement.

- Feedback mechanisms provide continuous learning and adaptation, which improves the effectiveness of somatic treatments for elders.

IX. Case Studies and Success Stories

- Real-world examples and testimonies demonstrate the benefits of somatic therapy for elders, emphasizing its ability to promote healing and improve quality of life.

Encouragement for Seniors to Embrace Somatic Healing

Encourage elders to embrace somatic healing by emphasizing the transformative advantages of therapies such as Somatic Experiencing (SE) and yoga. Seniors might be encouraged to investigate these methods to improve overall well-being, addressing physical and mental difficulties. By highlighting the benign nature of somatic techniques and their ability to release buried trauma, seniors can be encouraged to believe that healing is attainable at any age.

Creating a supportive and nurturing environment where elders feel empowered to explore their bodies and emotions is critical for instilling a sense of safety and trust. Finally, by embracing somatic healing, seniors can regain energy, connection, and joy in their daily lives, thus improving their overall quality of life as they age. Here are some encouraging points for seniors to embrace somatic therapy:

- Prioritize well-being through somatic exercises and mindfulness techniques to enhance overall quality of life.
- Address physical, emotional, and psychological challenges comprehensively by considering the interconnectedness of mind, body, and spirit.
- Explore gentle and accessible somatic exercises suitable for all fitness levels and mobility restrictions, including breathwork, mindful movement, and relaxation techniques.
- Seniors can reconnect with their bodies and actively participate in the healing process by practicing mindful movement and tuning into bodily sensations.
- Seniors find encouragement and support in community settings, offering somatic healing practices and fostering a sense of belonging and camaraderie.
- Seniors experience profound positive changes in physical health, emotional well-being, and overall vitality by embracing somatic healing and tapping into the innate capacity for healing.

Resources for Further Exploration

Here are some resources for you so you can further explore somatic therapy and gain a deeper understanding of its principles and practices. You can also explore them to get rid of any confusion, learn about the various exercises and techniques, and gain valuable insights into the application for healing and personal growth.

1. Somatic Therapy: Understanding The Mind-Body Connection

2. (PDF) 'A Brief History of Somatic Practices and Dance: Historical Development of the Field of Somatic Education and its Relationship to Dance

3. A Comprehensive Guide to Somatic Therapy | Everyday Health

4. A Guide: What Is Somatic Therapy?

5. Types and Uses of Somatic Trauma Therapy.

6. 10 Somatic Exercises To Release Pent-Up Emotions - BetterMe

7. 10 Somatic Interventions Explained — Integrative Psychotherapy Mental Health Blog

8. Somatic Techniques for Stress and Anxiety

9. Eight (8) Simple Breathing Exercises for Older Adults

10. Getting Started with Mindful Movement

11. Somatic experiencing: using interoception and proprioception as core elements of trauma therapy

12. 29 Best Group Therapy Activities for Supporting Adults

References

Araminta. (2021, December 24). 5 Benefits of Somatic Therapy. Khiron Clinics. https://khironclinics.com/blog/5-benefits-of-somatic-therapy/#:~:text=Conclusion

Atinga, A., Shekkeris, A., Fertleman, M., Batrick, N., Kashef, E., & Dick, E. (2018). Trauma in the elderly patient. The British Journal of Radiology, 91(1087), 20170739. https://doi.org/10.1259/bjr.20170739

Author, M. (2021, December 20). Somatic Therapy: Benefits, Types, Principles & More. Mantra Care. https://mantracare.org/therapy/therapy-types/somatic-therapy/

Bleser, G., Steffen, D., Weber, M., Hendeby, G., Stricker, D., Fradet, L., Marin, F., Ville, N., & Carré, F. (2013). A personalized exercise trainer for the elderly. Journal of Ambient Intelligence and Smart Environments, 5(6), 547–562. https://doi.org/10.3233/ais-130234

Braga, R. J., & Petrides, G. (2007). Terapias somáticas para transtornos psiquiátricos resistentes ao tratamento. Revista Brasileira de Psiquiatria, 29(suppl 2), S77–S84. https://doi.org/10.1590/s1516-44462007000600007

Conley, G. (2019, September 8). Breath and Movement Coordination. MamasteFit. https://mamastefit.com/breath-and-movement-coordination/

Cronkleton, E. (2019, April 9). 10 Breathing Techniques. Healthline; Healthline Media. https://www.healthline.com/health/breathing-exercise#takeaway

D. Metzl, J., M.D., & Barrow, K. (2017, April 14). The 9-Minute Strength Workout. The New York Times. https://www. nytimes.com/article/strength-training-plyometrics.html

Dallaway, N., Leo, S., & Ring, C. (2022). How am I doing? Performance feedback mitigates effects of mental fatigue on endurance exercise performance. Psychology of Sport and Exercise, 102210. https://doi.org/10.1016/j. psychsport.2022.102210

Deasy, H. (2014). Freedom to move, freedom to stop: A somatic approach to empowerment in community dance. Dance, Movement & Spiritualities, 1(1), 123–141. https://doi. org/10.1386/dmas.1.1.123_1

Drake, K. (2021, June 15). 3 Deep Breathing Exercises to Ease Anxiety. Psych Central. https://psychcentral.com/anxiety/ reduce-your-anxiety-this-minute-3-different-types-of-deep-breathing#about-deep-breathing

Dugan, R. (24 C.E., February 2). The Importance of Healing Past Trauma for Wellbeing. Www.linkedin.com; Rosemary Dugan. https://www.linkedin.com/pulse/importance-healing-past-trauma-wellbeing-rosemary-dugan-wstkc/?trk=article-ssr-frontend-pulse_more-articles_related-content-card

Eddy, Martha. (2009, June). A Brief History of Somatic Practices and Dance: Historical Development of the Field of Somatic Education and its Relationship to Dance. ReserchGate. https:// www.researchgate.net/publication/249920030 'A Brief History of Somatic Practices and Dance Historical Development of the Field of Somatic Education and its Relationship to Dance/citation/download

Eliaz, I. (2011, June 8). Why Stress Management Is So

Important For Your Health. Mindbodygreen. https://www.mindbodygreen.com/articles/why-stress-management-is-so-important-for-your-health

Eva. (2020, April 10). A Guided Sequence for Mindful Movement Meditation | PDF | Meditation | Mindfulness. Scribd. https://www.scribd.com/document/455873993/Mindful-Movement-Meditation

Fowler, P. (2018, January 11). Breathing techniques for stress relief. WebMD. https://www.webmd.com/balance/stress-management/stress-relief-breathing-techniques

Granero-Jiménez, J., López-Rodríguez, M. M., Dobarrio-Sanz, I., & Cortés-Rodríguez, A. E. (2022). Influence of Physical Exercise on Psychological Well-Being of Young Adults: A Quantitative Study. International Journal of Environmental Research and Public Health, 19(7). https://doi.org/10.3390/ijerph19074282

HCA DEV. (2019, April 4). 6 Effects of Stress on Aging Adults. Home Care Assistance of Toronto. https://www.torontohomecareassistance.ca/stress-effects-on-elderly/

Heydlauf, J. (2023, April 6). Signs and Causes of Stress in Seniors | | Grand Oaks Blog. Grand Oaks. https://www.grandoaksdc.org/common-signs-and-causes-of-stress-in-seniors/

Hughes, D. C., Ellefsen, S., & Baar, K. (2017). Adaptations to Endurance and Strength Training. Cold Spring Harbor Perspectives in Medicine, 8(6), a029769. https://doi.org/10.1101/cshperspect.a029769

lyra Team. (2023, September 12). Recognizing the Signs of

Emotional Trauma in Adults. Lyra Health. https://www.lyrahealth.com/blog/signs-emotional-trauma-in-adults/

Khanzan, I. (2019). Biofeedback and mindfulness in everyday life: Practical solutions for improving your health and performance. Psycnet.apa.org. https://psycnet.apa.org/record/2019-35696-000

KIM. (2020, September 25). 5 Reasons Elderly People Become Stressed. Home Care Assistance of Amarillo, TX. https://www.homecareassistanceamarillo.com/sources-of-stress-for-aging-adults/

Kristin McGee. (2018, November 12). mindbodygreen. Mindbodygreen. https://www.mindbodygreen.com/articles/the-11-major-types-of-yoga-explained-simply

Krouse, L. (2023, August 11). A Comprehensive Guide to Somatic Therapy. EverydayHealth.com. https://www.everydayhealth.com/emotional-health/somatic-therapy/

Krouse, L. (2023, August 11). A Comprehensive Guide to Somatic Therapy. EverydayHealth.com. https://www.everydayhealth.com/emotional-health/somatic-therapy/

Lambert, M. I. (2016). General Adaptations to Exercise: Acute Versus Chronic and Strength Versus Endurance Training. Exercise and Human Reproduction, 93–100. https://doi.org/10.1007/978-1-4939-3402-7_6

Lonczak, H. (2021, May 5). Geriatric Therapy: How to Help Older Adults With Depression. PositivePsychology.com. https://positivepsychology.com/geriatric-therapy-older-adults-depression/

Lucini, D., & Pagani, M. (2021). Exercise Prescription to Foster Health and Well-Being: A Behavioral Approach to Transform Barriers into Opportunities. International Journal of Environmental Research and Public Health, 18(3), 968. https://doi.org/10.3390/ijerph18030968

Majsiak, B., & Young, C. (2022, June 23). 5 Ways to Practice Breath-Focused Meditation | Everyday Health. EverydayHealth.com. https://www.everydayhealth.com/alternative-health/living-with/ways-practice-breath-focused-meditation/

Martens, N. L. (2022). Yoga Interventions Involving Older Adults: Integrative Review. Journal of Gerontological Nursing, 48(2), 43–52. https://doi.org/10.3928/00989134-20220110-05

Marturana, A. (2022, June 13). The 21 Best Stretching Exercises for Better Flexibility. SELF. https://www.self.com/gallery/essential-stretches-slideshow

Moore, M. (2022, July 25). 6 Benefits of Stress Management. Psych Central. https://psychcentral.com/stress/the-benefits-of-stress-management#heart-rate

NHS. (2021, February 2). Breathing exercises for stress. Nhs. uk. https://www.nhs.uk/mental-health/self-help/guides-tools-and-activities/breathing-exercises-for-stress/

Nothaft, D. (2023, April 19). Is it trauma or something else? How to recognize trauma in others. USA TODAY. https://www.usatoday.com/story/life/health-wellness/2023/04/19/how-recognize-trauma-others-five-signs-plus-ptsd-symptoms/11680701002/

OfferingTree. https://www.offeringtree.com/blog/2-person-yoga-poses/

Orenstein, B. (2019, February 21). 8 Yoga Poses for Beginners and Their Benefits. EverydayHealth.com. https://www.everydayhealth.com/fitness-pictures/yoga-poses-for-beginners.aspx

Othership, & reserved, A. right. (2021, October 17). Breathwork for Healing Trauma: 3 Popular Techniques + Benefits. Www.othership.us. https://www.othership.us/resources/breathwork-for-healing-trauma

Parrott, M. (2016, April 25). Transitional exercises keep up pace between reps. Arkansas Online. https://www.nwaonline.com/news/2016/apr/25/transitional-exercises-keep-up-pace-bet/

Ph.D, M. M. (2023, November 21). 29 Best Group Therapy Activities for Supporting Adults. PositivePsychology.com. https://positivepsychology.com/group-therapy-activities/

Pizer, A. (2013, August 13). Must-Know Yoga Poses for Beginners. Verywell Fit; Verywellfit. https://www.verywellfit.com/essential-yoga-poses-for-beginners-3566747

Poet, J. (2019, October 18). Flow Yoga Sequences for Beginners. Healthy Life Essex. https://healthylifeessex.co.uk/2019/10/flow-yoga-sequences-for-beginners/

Porrey, M. (2024, February 1). Types and Uses of Somatic Trauma Therapy. Verywell Health. https://www.verywellhealth.com/somatic-trauma-therapy-5218970#:~:text=Through%20the%20use%20of%20movement

Porteous, B., & Sebouhian. (2022, March 4). What is somatic therapy and why is it perfect for trauma recovery? Www.linkedin.com. https://www.linkedin.com/pulse/what-somatic-therapy-why-perfect-trauma-recovery-

Preskorn, S. H., & Burke, M. (1992). Somatic therapy for major depressive disorder: selection of an antidepressant. The Journal of Clinical Psychiatry, 53 Suppl, 5–18. https://europepmc.org/article/med/1522080

Quinn, D. (2023a, May 25). Somatic Therapy: Understanding The Mind-Body Connection. Sandstone Care. https://www.sandstonecare.com/blog/somatic-therapy/#:~:text=Somatic%20therapy%2C%20also%20referred%20to

Quinn, D. (2023b, August 3). Types of Trauma: The 7 Most Common Types & Their Impacts. Sandstone Care. https://www.sandstonecare.com/blog/types-of-trauma/

Ra McComas, V. (2023, October 16). The Essence of Somatic Therapy: Mind, Body, and Beyond. Www.linkedin.com. https://www.linkedin.com/pulse/essence-somatic-therapy-mind-body-beyond-vishnu-ra-mccomas-qlp3c

Rae Ackerman, L. (2023, December 18). Benefits of Mindful Breathing Exercises for Stress Relief. Www.linkedin.com. https://www.linkedin.com/pulse/benefits-mindful-breathing-exercises-stress-relief-do8ec?trk=public_post

Rasmussen, P., Milana, M., Vatrella, S., & Larson, A. (2021). Aalborg Universitet Knowledge Production, Public Media and Adult Education and Learning How the OECD'S PIAAC survey enters the press discourse in Italy and Denmark. https://vbn.aau.dk/ws/portalfiles/portal/456089724/2021_CASAE_Proceedings.pdf#page=429

Robinson, A. (2020, July 17). How to do Yoga Team Building Activities in 2024. Teambuilding.com. https://teambuilding.com/blog/team-building-yoga

Robinson, L. (2019, May 2). Relaxation Techniques for Stress Relief. HelpGuide.org. https://www.helpguide.org/articles/

stress/relaxation-techniques-for-stress-relief.htm

Rothberg, R. (2014). Application of somatic interventions in clinical practice Application of somatic interventions in clinical practice. https://scholarworks.smith.edu/cgi/viewcontent.cgi?article=1807&context=theses

Salamon, M. (2023, July 7). What is somatic therapy? Harvard Health. https://www.health.harvard.edu/blog/what-is-somatic-therapy-202307072951

Salisbury, J., Huberty, J., Sullivan, M., Curtin, N., & Sarah Ellen Braun. (2022). Summary of Mindful Movement Sequences. Springer EBooks, 111–184. https://doi.org/10.1007/978-3-030-91062-4_13

Schöne, B., Gruber, T., Graetz, S., Bernhof, M., & Malinowski, P. (2018). Mindful breath awareness meditation facilitates efficiency gains in brain networks: A steady-state visually evoked potentials study. Scientific Reports, 8(1). https://doi.org/10.1038/s41598-018-32046-5

Sinead. (2022, July 26). 15 Fun 2 Person Yoga Poses To Do With Friends | OfferingTree.

Staff, M. (2023, February 7). Getting Started with Mindful Movement. Mindful. https://www.mindful.org/getting-started-with-mindful-movement/#:~:text=Mindful%20movement%20can%20help%20you

Stora, J. B. (2023). The Psychosomatic Therapy Casebook : Stories from the Intersection of Mind and Body. Www.torrossa.com, 1–224. https://www.torrossa.com/en/resources/an/5624728

Straussner, S. L. A., & Calnan, A. J. (2014). Trauma Through the Life Cycle: A Review of Current Literature. Clinical Social Work Journal, 42(4), 323–335. https://doi.org/10.1007/

s10615-014-0496-z

Sutton, J. (2021, December 20). 7 Stress-Relief Breathing Exercises for Calming Your Mind. PositivePsychology.com. https://positivepsychology.com/breathing-exercises-for-stress-relief/

Thorgal256. (2020, January 30). Somatic Experiencing Has Been Liberating Me. Reddit. https://www.reddit.com/r/SomaticExperiencing/comments/evskot/comment/ffz1flp/?utm_source=share&utm_medium=web3x&utm_name=web3xcss&utm_term=1&utm_content=share_button

Trewick, N., Neumann, D. L., & Hamilton, K. (2022). Effect of affective feedback and competitiveness on performance and the psychological experience of exercise within a virtual reality environment. PLOS ONE, 17(6), e0268460. https://doi.org/10.1371/journal.pone.0268460

Vogels, S. (2019, July 17). Somatization: Understanding the Mind-Body Connection | Kelty Mental Health. Keltymentalhealth.ca. https://keltymentalhealth.ca/blog/2019/07/somatization-understanding-mind-body-connection

Wackerhage, H., & Schoenfeld, B. J. (2021). Personalized, Evidence-Informed Training Plans and Exercise Prescriptions for Performance, Fitness and Health. Sports Medicine, 51(9), 1805–1813. https://doi.org/10.1007/s40279-021-01495-w

Zuda, T. (2022, June 8). 4 Person Yoga Poses To Try With A Group – Zud

Yoga. ZUDA YOGA. https://zudayoga.com/4-person-yoga-poses-to-try-with-a-group